PAEDIATRICS AND BLOOD TRANSFUSION

DEVELOPMENTS IN HEMATOLOGY AND IMMUNOLOGY

VOLUME 2

1. Lijnen HR, Collen D and Verstraete M: Synthetic Substrates in Clinical Blood Coagulation Assays. 1980. ISBN 90-247-2409-0

Series ISBN 90-247-2432-5

PAEDIATRICS AND BLOOD TRANSFUSION

Proceedings of the Fifth Annual Symposium on Blood Transfusion, Groningen 1980 organized by the Red Cross Bloodbank Groningen-Drenthe

edited by

C.TH. SMIT SIBINGA,
P.C. DAS,
Red Cross Bloodbank Groningen-Drenthe

and

J.O. FORFAR
Department of Child Life and Health,
University of Edinburgh

1982

MARTINUS NIJHOFF PUBLISHERS
THE HAGUE / BOSTON / LONDON

Distributors

for the United States and Canada
Kluwer Boston, Inc.
190 Old Derby Street
Hingham, MA 02043
USA

for all other countries
Kluwer Academic Publishers Group
Distribution Center
P.O. Box 322
3300 AH Dordrecht
The Netherlands

Library of Congress Cataloging in Publication Data

Symposium on Blood Transfusion (5th : 1980 :
Groningen, Netherlands)
Paediatrics and blood transfusion.

(Developments in hematology ; v. 2)
1. Erythroblastosis fetalis--Congresses.
2. Blood--Transfusion--Congresses. 3. Pediatric hematology--Congresses. I. Smit Sibinga, C. Th.
II. Das, P. C. III. Forfar, John O. IV. Stichting Rode Kruis Bloedbank Groningen/Drente. V. Title.
VI. Series. [DNLM: 1. Blood transfusion--In infancy and childhood--Congresses. 2. Erythroblastosis, Fetal--Therapy--Congresses. W1 DE997VZH v. 2 / WH 425 S989 1980p]

RJ270.S94 1980 618.92'15 81-22437
AACR2

ISBN-13: 978-94-009-7522-4 e-ISBN-13: 978-94-009-7520-0
DOI: 10.1007/978-94-009-7520-0

FOREWORD

The practice of transfusing blood started at the bedside but over the last few decades blood transfusion has become more and more a laboratory directed discipline. The emphasis on serology and laboratory controlled measures has made blood transfusion safer and more effective, but laboratory and clinical aspects of the discipline have tended to become increasingly separated. As a result of this separation clinical developments in blood transfusion may not have derived full benefit from the knowledge accrued in blood transfusion services. Over the last five years the Red Cross Blood Bank Groningen-Drenthe has organised yearly symposia with a clinical theme in order to bring blood banks and clinicians closer together.

Many of the recent major advances in clinical medicine have been based on developments in blood transfusion practice. This is certainly true for paediatric medicine. For instance, in paediatric oncology, including leukemia, cell separator programmes have made available new forms of support. Further, blood component therapy has provided an effective means of control in some of the bleeding disorders of children. Some of these topics are discussed in this symposium dealing with intensive care.

Haemolytic disease of the newborn and exchange transfusion are other aspects of intensive care. Our purpose in dealing with them was twofold. Firstly, in earlier days, the greater prevalence of haemolytic disease of the newborn meant that exchange transfusion had to be carried out in many different hospitals. The last five years, however, have seen a significant reduction in the size of the problem so that exchange transfusion will now have to be carried out in fewer centres on a regional or supra-regional basis if an appropriate degree of skill and expertise is to be maintained. It thus seemed appropriate to take the opportunity presented by a workshop and symposium to document the knowledge, expertise and experience that are available about a specialty on which many will have to be informed but which few will practise.

Secondly, the suitability and availability of blood for exchange transfusion are current problems in the developed countries of the world.

Most paediatric units use citrate-phosphate-dextrose (CPD) anticoagulated blood for exchange transfusion. CPD is the anticoagulant routinely employed in blood banks and CPD blood is used for the separation and preparation of multiple blood products and components. In a few paediatric centres, but a few only, fresh heparinised blood is considered necessary for exchange transfusion. The pros and cons of these two methods of anticoagulation for blood used in exchange transfusion is a subject on which this meeting deliberated.

In the wider field of blood usage transfusion of blood, as opposed to the selective use of blood components and blood products, tends to receive a disproportionately large share of attention. Some of the classical texts on blood transfusion devote much attention to transfusion but very little to topics such as blood component therapy and haematological supportive therapy for host defence. There appear to be gaps between the knowledge that is available on blood usage and the practical application of that knowledge. It is the object of this Workshop and Symposium to try to bridge these gaps within paediatric medicine.

P. C. Das
John Forfar
C. Th. Smit Sibinga

ACKNOWLEDGEMENTS

This publication has been made possible through the support of Travenol, which is gratefully acknowledged.
Tape transcription and typewriting: Judy Fagelston, London.

OPENING ADDRESS

K. KNOL

It was a good idea of the organisers of this symposium of the Red Cross Bloodbank Groningen-Drenthe to dedicate this Fifth Symposium to the subject of "Paediatrics and bloodtransfusion". In some parts of the Netherlands each fifth anniversary is called a crown-year and the person concerned gets special attention on that day. As president of the Dutch Paediatric Association I feel honoured that on the occasion of this first crown-year of the Bloodbank Symposium the benefits of bloodtransfusion, or the transfusion of blood components in children's disease will draw the attention of all participants. As in so many fields of medicine, advancement in knowledge and technique has been impressive during the last years.

When I was preparing this short opening address my thoughts went back to the days of my own period of residency in the Paediatric Department in Groningen. I do not consider myself an old man, who is looking back to the old times, but I cannot resist recalling that time some twenty-five years ago. If we decided to give a transfusion, whole blood was ordered and control consisted of putting together a tiny drop of erythrocytes with a few tiny drops of A, B and Rhesus D antibody solution taken from some tiny bottles. When looked at through the microscope there were two possibilities. The erythrocytes floated free, which always was a very nice sight, and the transfusion could be started; or they clotted and we had to order another bottle; or, finally, we had to call for Dr. Kaars Sijpesteijn, now head of the Bloodgrouping Laboratory, to get us out of trouble. Things have certainly changed during the last two decades! Thinking about these changes, I think we can congratulate the organisers of this symposium, Dr. Smit Sibinga and Dr. Das, in advance on their success in bringing together such an impressive group of moderators and speakers for the various sessions of the symposium and workshop.

I will not mention them all now. Their names can be found in the programme and the list of participants. I will make an exception for two: Professor Forfar, professor of paediatrics in Edinburgh, whose Textbook of Paediatrics is a guide for so many students of medicine and paediatricians and who has consented to chair the symposium, and Dr. Birger Broman of Stockholm, whom we are very glad to have with us today, and who, in his thesis in 1944 introduced the now well-known collective name of "morbus haemolyticus neonatorum".

Dr. Smit Sibinga told me that one of the origins of this symposium is the discussion about the use of certain anticoagulants in exchange transfusions in newborns. In the clinical situation I now and then overhear bits of these discussions. Not being an expert in this field myself - not by far - I will make only one remark about the subject: I think it is extremely important that workers in the clinical field and laboratory doctors really listen to each other's experiences and arguments with regard to this absorbing item. With this in mind I express the expectation that this workshop and symposium will be fruitful and successful.

Prof. K. Knol, MD,PhD
President, Dutch Paediatric Association

CONTENTS

INVITED SPEAKERS

Bennebroek Gravenhorst, J., MD, PhD
- professor of obstetrics
  Department of Obstetrics & Gynaecology
  University of Leiden, The Netherlands

Broman, B., MD, PhD
- Karolinska Hospital Blood Centre
  Stockholm, Sweden

Bijlmer, R.P.G.M., MD, PhD
- consultant paediatrician
  Wilhemina Kinder Ziekenhuis
  University of Utrecht, The Netherlands

Das, P.C., MD, PhD, MRC Path.
- Red Cross Bloodbank Groningen-Drenthe
  Groningen, The Netherlands

Eernisse, J.G., MD, PhD
- medical director
  University Hospital Bloodbank
  Leiden, The Netherlands

Forfar, J.O., MC,BSc,MD,FRCPE,FRCP,RCH
chairman
- professor of paediatrics
  Department of Child Life and Health
  University of Edinburgh, Scotland

Garratty, G., FIMLS
moderator
- scientific director
  American Red Cross Blood Services
  Orange County Service, Los Angeles
  California, U.S.A.

Hekker, A.C., PhD
- Department of Microbiology
  National Institute of Public Health
  Bilthoven, The Netherlands

Holman, C.A., MB, FRCP, FRCPath
- consultant haematologist
  Rhesus Immunisation Unit
  Lewisham Hospital, London, England

Israëls, S.P., MD, PhD
moderator
- medical director
  Red Cross Bloodbank Amsterdam
  The Netherlands

Kerr, M.M., MD, FRCP, DCH - consultant paediatrician
The Queen Mother's Hospital
Glasgow, Scotland

Khalifa, A.S., MD, PhD - professor of pediatrics
Department of Paediatrics
Ain Shams University
Cairo, Egypt

Koning, J. de, MD, PhD - consultant paediatrician
Department of Paediatrics
University of Leiden, The Netherlands

Lockyer, J.W., PhD - South West Regional Blood Transfusion
Laboratories, Southmead
Bristol, England

Overby, L.R., PhD - director experimental biology
Abbott Diagnostic Division
North Chicago, Illinois, U.S.A.

Postma, A., MD - consultant paediatrician
Division of Paediatric Oncology
Department of Paediatrics
University of Groningen, The Netherlands

Reerink-Brongers, E.E., MD, PhD
- Central Laboratory of the Dutch Red Cross
Amsterdam, The Netherlands

Roberton, N.R.C., MA,MB,BCHR,FRCP
moderator - consultant paediatrician
Department of Paediatrics
Addenbrooke's Hospital, Cambridge, England

Ruys, J.H., MD, PhD - associate professor of paediatrics
moderator
Department of Paediatrics
University of Leiden, The Netherlands

Smallenbroek, A.J.G. - Pharmacy Department
University of Groningen, The Netherlands

Turner, Th.L., MB, ChB, MRCP - consultant paediatrician
Department of Paediatrics
The Hull Royal Infirmary, England

I. HISTORICAL PERSPECTIVES OF HAEMOLYTIC DISEASE OF THE NEWBORN

B. BROMAN

The introduction of blood typing for Rh in Sweden in 1943 was a thrilling event.

We learned about the discovery of the Rh factor from an article in the British Medical Journal and about the significance of the Rh antigen in familial erythroblastosis neonatorum. No Rh tests had at that time been carried out in Sweden. But, with the world at war we were unable to obtain specific Rh test sera from abroad.

The following, which quickly led us to our goal, was therefore chosen as a suitable starting point for our work. Blood samples were taken from a number of mothers who had had children recently treated on the diagnosis of icterus gravis neonatorum. At the same time, we immunised six guineapigs with blood cells from macaque rhesus monkeys.

The experiments to obtain a human anti-Rh serum succeeded with our third patient. Her serum contained an atypical irregular agglutinin which agglutinated between 80% and 90% of tested A and O blood cells, irrespective of their group in the MN or P systems. Immediately after this we were able to obtain a further serum with an atypical irregular agglutinin for yet another mother of an erythroblastotic child. As this later serum had the same reactions as the former there was good reason to suppose that an anti-Rh agglutinin was the common factor. These results were substantiated when sera were subsequently obtained from the guineapigs and three of these agglutinated red cells in the same manner as the two human sera.

The patients who provided the suspected anti-Rh agglutinin belonged to group A. Therefore the serum could not be used for testing B or AB cells without removing the anti-B. At that time we had no B cells known to be Rh negative.

We took random samples of B blood and absorbed the A sera which contained anti-Rh. We showed that B Rh positive cells too were suitable for this purpose. At a low temperature, the anti-B was readily absorbed by B cells in a very short time. On the other hand, most of the anti-Rh remained because even Rh positive cells, when untreated, are very poor absorbers of Rh antibodies, especially in brief periods at a low temperature. Thus we obtained human anti-Rh test sera for use with all ABO groups.

I should point out that at that time the only generally used method for agglutinating red cells with test sera involved the use of saline medium. We did not then know of methods involving the use of antiglobulin, or of enzyme treated cells, or the method of adding albumin to the test. Nor had Wiener's insensitive blocking test to show IgG antibodies been invented.

As a result, many questions arose when we studied serum from patients with saline method to show Rh antibodies and when we typed the red blood cells for Rh factor with pure Rh agglutinins (i.e. IgM antibodies). The use of both human anti-Rh sera and anti-rhesus serum from guineapigs confused the situation still further.

We found, independently of Fisk and Ford in the U.S. that almost all newborn infants' red cells reacted positively to anti-rhesus serum from guineapigs. With human anti-Rh sera only 85% of the bloods from infants reacted positively. We could not explain why this happened, but drew the conclusion that anti-rhesus serum from guineapigs was useless for bloodtyping for the Rh factor in newborns.

Since that time, Philip Levine has shown that anti-rhesus serum from guineapigs has an antibody against a factor other than the human factor which is responsible for most cases of haemolytic disease of the newborn. I therefore never use the word "rhesus" to denote the new human bloodgroup found in 1939. Rhesus should be used to denote an antigen found in the red cells of the rhesus macacus monkey. The human Rh factor is not a rhesus antigen, but a very complex antigen found in human red cells which can be detected only with human anti-Rh sera of different specificities, and not with anti-rhesus serum. The name Rh only refers to the contribution which the anti-rhesus serum from guineapigs once made to the discovery of the human Rh factor.

The next point which threw doubt on the accuracy of the theory that Rh immunisation was the cause of haemolytic disease of the newborn was the following. In many cases of the most severe erythroblastosis - even those with a typical familial history of sick siblings - an obviously weak agglutination was often found when the red cells from the newborn were tested with anti-Rh agglutinin. In those cases it was often impossible to show Rh agglutinin in the serum of the Rh negative mother. If we consider the case of a seriously ill infant with an apparently weak Rh antigen, whose mother has very weak, or no, Rh antibodies in her serum we might well doubt that that child is ill because of Rh immunisation. Now, of course, we know about IgG Rh antibodies which can cause blocking of Rh-sites on the infant's red cells. We also have methods to show IgG antibodies both on the infant's red cells and in the mother's serum: specifically enzyme and antiglobulin methods and autoanalysers.

During the years that followed, when Rh serology was established and put into practice in the treatment of pregnant women and in blood transfusions, the search began for more effective treatment of newborn infants with haemolytic disease. A simple transfusion of Rh negative blood to the infant was of little use. The real answer was an exchange transfusion - often multiple transfusions - to the newborn; the death rate then went down from more than 50% to less than 3%.

In Sweden we first developed these methods of treatment in Stockholm and were soon able to show that Diamond's catheter technique for exchange transfusions gave good results. About one-third of the sick infants were managed without transfusions. Later on the treatment was extended to nine large regional hospitals throughout the country.

The latest advance in managing the disease is to prevent Rh immunisation by prophylactic treatment. We administer 250 - 300 micrograms of anti-D intramascularly during the first few days after delivery as well as after various interventions, such as abortion, amniocentesis and other operations which may cause transplacental haemorrhage. Intrauterine transfusions to the baby and prophylactic treatment routinely with anti-D during pregnancy are given in only a few hospitals in Sweden. The same applies to repeated plasma exchange transfusions of pregnant strongly-immunised women. Some researchers have noted that such intensive plasma exchanges for the purpose of reducing the maternal anti-D concentration have produced adverse effects.

However that may be, the elucidation of the pathogenesis of this disease, the introduction of proper treatment and the discovery of an effective prophylaxis against D-immunisation within the space of twenty-five years all add up to an unusual achievement in the sphere of haemolytic disease of the newborn. The numerous researchers in various English-speaking countries who have been engaged in this work deserve our admiration.

1. THE SEROLOGICAL INVESTIGATION OF HAEMOLYTIC DISEASE OF THE NEWBORN

G.G. GARRATTY

Haemolytic Disease of the Newborn (HDN) is a condition in the fetus and neonate in which the lifespan of the infant's red cells is shortened by the action of maternal antibodies. These antibodies must be capable of crossing the placenta and thus are always IgG. They are usually formed as a result of pregnancy or previous bloodtransfusion. Theoretically, any IgG antibody can cause HDN, but many factors affect its clinical significance; the most important factors are listed in Table I.

TABLE I

FACTORS AFFECTING THE CLINICAL SIGNIFICANCE OF IgG ANTIBODIES IN HDN

1. Presence, or strength, of appropriate antigen on infant's red cells
2. Strength of maternal antibody
3. Inhibitory effect of antigen present on infant's tissues and in body fluids
4. IgG subclass of antibody
5. Rate of transfer of antibody across placenta

It is convenient to classify the IgG antibodies causing HDN into three main groups:

1. Anti-D
2. "Others" (anti-c, -E, -K, etc.)
3. ABO (anti-A, -B, A,B)

PRENATAL TESTING

At the initial prenatal visit, all women should have the following tests performed: (1) ABO group; (2) Rh(D) group; if Rh negative, then a D^u test should be performed; (3) serum tested for unexpected antibodies. The results of these tests will provide useful information with regard not only to the possibility of HDN occurring but also to any problems that may occur if bloodtransfusion is required.

Rh negative women whose sera contain no unexpected antibodies should have their sera examined again at approximately 28-30 weeks. If no antibodies are detected at this time, then no further prenatal testing need be made.

When unexpected antibodies are detected, they should be identified. If screening tests include testing at room temperature, then the antibodies most commonly detected may have no clinical significance; e.g., anti-I and anti-Lewis. It is recommended that all screening, and indeed compatibility testing, be carried out only at 37 C.

Methods of antibody screening vary, but are usually similar to the methods used for compatibility testing in that particular institution. I would use two separate reagent red cell screening samples that cover all common blood group antigens. The patient's sera are tested against these red cells suspended in low ionic strength saline (LISS), at 37 C.[1,8] Two volumes of the patient's serum are added to two volumes of 2% LISS suspended red cells and incubated at 37C for 15 mins. The tubes are centrifuged; inspected for agglutination; washed with normal saline four times, and an antiglobulin test performed. Some workers recommend using enzyme-treated red cells, either alone, or in addition to, non-enzyme-treated red cells. It certainly is possible to detect weaker antibodies, (e.g., Rh) earlier in the pregnancy when enzyme-treated red cells or autoanalyser methods are used, but it is rare for these antibodies not to be detected by the LISS method towards the end of the pregnancy. It would seem very unlikely that such antibodies would cause harm to the fetus before they became detectable by the LISS procedure. There appears still to be disagreement as to whether Rh immune globulin (Rh IG) should be given to an

Rh negative mother whose serum contains an enzyme-only or autoanalyser-only reactive anti-D. Theoretically, once the mother has started producing antibody, Rh IG will have no effect, but as it causes no harm to the patient, many workers would prefer to give the mother Rh IG following delivery of an Rh (D) positive infant. Some workers have expressed concern that if enzyme-treated red cells are used routinely, especially by inexperienced personnel, an increased proportion of clinically insignificant antibodies may be detected, (e.g., anti-Lewis), leading to reporting of a positive antibody screen and Rh IG being withheld.

I personally used and recommended the use of enzyme-treated red cells in antenatal screening for many years, before using LISS, but can appreciate some of these fears that have been expressed by some workers in the USA. I would have no hesitation in recommending their usage by experienced laboratory workers who can interpret the results correctly for the attending physicians.

Approximately 2-4% of patients' sera will contain unexpected antibodies. More antibodies may be detected if a cooler room temperature phase is used, but if reacting only at that temperature, these will be clinically insignificant.[11]

The pattern of specificities observed has been changing over the last two decades. This has been due to increased blood transfusion and the use of Rh prophylaxis. Giblett[9] reported that 70% of the clinically significant antibodies detected in hospital patients in 1956-7 were anti-D, whereas in 1974-5 only 32% were anti-D and many more of the Rh negative patients whose sera contained anti-D also contained non-Rh antibodies (e.g., anti-K, $-Jk^a$, $-Fy^a$). Spielman and Seidl[23] did not find such a difference in their study from 1965-72, where pregnant women were examined separately from blood recipients. In their study, serum from 2.85% of 16,643 pregnant women contained antibodies reactive at 37 C. Eighty percent of these sera contained anti-D. Three percent of these anti-D-containing-sera also contained non-Rh antibodies (e.g., -K, $-Fy^a$, $-Jk^a$). Only 2% of the antibody-containing-sera from pregnant women, compared with 25% of female blood recipients, contained clinically significant antibodies without anti-D being present. As Rh prophylaxis only gained momentum after 1968, it is possible that a more current study would yield different statistics.

Table II lists the antibodies that have been described as being associated with HDN. Some of the reports were poorly documented clinically. For instance, some reports proved that the positive direct antiglobulin test was due

TABLE II

ANTIGENS THAT HAVE BEEN INVOLVED IN HDN

Common Antigens		High Frequency Antigens		Low Frequency Antigens	
c	Fy^a	At^a	k	Be^a	Js^a
C	Jk^a	Co^a	Kp^b(mild)	Bi	Kam(Far)
Ce	Jk^b	Di^b	Lan(mild)	By	Kp^a
D	K	Ge(mild)	Lu^b(?)	C^w	Mit
Do^a	Lu^a	Hr_o	LW	C^x	Mt^a
e	M	Hy	P, P_1, p^k	Di^a	Mull
E	N	Jr^a(mild)	U	Evans	Mur
f(?)	S	Js^b	Yt^a	E^w	Rd
G	s			Far	Re^a
				Ga	R^N
				Go^a	Vw(Gr)
				Good	Wr^a
				Heibel	Zd
				Hil	Allen
				Ht^a	Joslin
				Hut	Kuhn
					Niemetz
					Reiter
					Sharp

Data taken mainly from Reference 21

to the maternal antibody, but there was little evidence that the sensitisation was causing a clinical problem.

If Unexpected Antibodies Are Detected

If unexpected antibodies are detected at 37 C and are present on Table II, then they should be titrated against red cells possessing the appropriate antigens. When titrations are performed, it is useful to record an agglutination score[1,14] as well as a titre. The serum should be frozen away so that it can be titrated in parallel against further samples from the same patient. Once antibody is detected, titrations are usually performed at least monthly. A change of titre of more than two tubes (over fourfold), or a score of more than 10, is a significant change, if the techniques are carefully standardised.

The principal value of antibody titrations is to identify those women who are candidates for amniocentesis. Titres of 8-32 or greater are usually an indication for amniocentesis. Antibody titration is generally not helpful in the prenatal management of ABO HDN.

If unexpected 37 C reacting antibodies are identified and they are not present on Table II, then it is useful to know their potential for causing HDN by determining whether they are IgG or IgM. This can be easily determined by adding 2-mercaptoethanol (2-ME) or dithiothreitol (DTT) to the patient's serum.[1,13] If reactions persist after treatment with these chemicals, then IgG antibodies can be presumed to be present (possibly together with IgM); if the reactions become negative, then the antibodies are probably IgM and will not cross the placenta. The patient's serum must, of course, be retested later in the pregnancy as the IgM antibodies might change into IgG.

TABLE III

RELATIVE STRENGTH OF ANTIGENS ON FETAL RED CELLS

	Antigen Strength	Blood Group System or Antigen
I	Well developed at birth	Diego Dombrock Duffy En^a Gerbich i Kell Kidd MNSsU Rh Scianna Yt^b
II	Present at birth - weaker than adult	ABH Lutheran P_1 Xg^a
III	Very weak or absent at birth	Chido I Lewis Sd^a Vel Yt^a

Data taken mainly from Reference 12

Some relatively commonly detected antibodies, such as anti-I, P_1, Le^a and Le^b, do not ever cause HDN and once identified, their immunoglobulin class does not need to be determined. Most fetal red cells have weak P_1 antigens and have very little, if any, detectable I, Le^a, or Le^b antigens; thus, even if the antibodies were to cross the placenta, they would not be expected to cause any immune red cell destruction. Table III lists the relative strength of blood group antigens on fetal red cells.

It is becoming increasingly common to give Rh(D) immunoglobulin (Rh IG) to Rh negative women following amniocentesis, and even during pregnancy; e.g.,at 28 weeks.[2] This anti-D can be readily detected in the patients' sera. When 300 μgs of anti-Rh(D) has been given, passive antibody is usually detectable by the antiglobulin test at a level of about 1:4 at 48 hours and 1:1 or 1:2 at six weeks and may be found by enzyme techniques up to six months later. When 4000-6000 μgs of anti-Rh(D) were injected by Pollack et al, passive antibody was detectable for 9-12 months. Passive antibody may be found even when there are still large numbers of circulating Rh positive cells.[17] The bloodbank must be notified that a patient has received Rh IG so that the serum screening and antibody titres can be interpreted correctly. Care must be taken that passive antibody present from an injection given prior to delivery is not mistaken for evidence of active immunisation and the post-delivery injection withheld.

<u>Phenotyping</u>

If anti-D is detected, it is useful to phenotype the father of the child. Knowing the probable genotype of the father is useful to the physician for advising the mother about future pregnancies and possibly assessing severity of disease if amniocentesis is not possible. If other antibodies are detected, then the mother should be phenotyped to prove she lacks the offending antigen and the father typed to assess the probability of the child possessing the antigen. For instance, Polesky[15] reported the data in Table IV. Only 14 of 59 patients whose husbands were typed for Kell were married to Kell positive men. A history of transfusion was obtained from almost half of those individuals married to Kell negatives. Since the histories were incomplete, it is highly probable that all of these women had received transfusions at one time. Thus, in those cases where the father is kk, both the physician and patient can be reassured that the baby will not be affected with HDN.

TABLE IV

INCIDENCE OF ANTI-KELL
IN 43,000 PRENATAL SERA *

Antibodies to Kell		Percentage known to have been transfused
Number of Women with anti-K	91	31
Husband - Kell type known	59	
Husband Kell Positive	14	14
Husband Kell Negative (kk)	45	44

*see Reference 15

NEONATAL TESTING

A sample of cord blood should be collected from every newborn and stored in the bloodbank at 4 C for at least seven days. The tube should be labelled with the mother's name, baby's identification, hospital number and date. Many hospitals perform a direct antiglobulin test on every sample, but I agree with others[3] that this is an unnecessary expense. If all samples are stored in the bloodbank refrigerator, then they are readily available for testing if the newborn develops signs and symptoms of HDN. If HDN is suspected, the following serological tests are performed: (1) ABO and Rh(D) type, and D^u testing if Rh(D) negative, on mother's and baby's blood; (2) direct antiglobulin test (DAT) on baby's red cells; (3) if DAT is positive, prepare an eluate from baby's red cells; (4) identify specificity of antibody in eluate from baby's red cells and in mother's serum.

ABO and Rh Grouping Problems: The ABO group of the baby should be based solely on the red cell tests as the baby's serum may contain maternal ABO antibodies. If the baby has received intrauterine transfusions of group O Rh negative blood, the cord sample may type clearly as a group O Rh negative, or show varying degrees of mixed field reactions with anti-A, anti-B or anti-Rh (i.e., detecting the infant's own A or B Rh positive red cells). Similarly, the DAT may show a mixed field reaction.

It may be difficult to obtain an accurate Rh typing on the baby with a strongly positive DAT. The result may be falsely negative because the Rh(D) sites are blocked by maternal antibody. If a mother is known to have Rh(D) antibodies and the baby is born with a strongly positive DAT and types as Rh negative, an error should be suspected. The baby's cells should be heated to 45 C for about 10 mins. along with a known Rh positive and negative control, and then retested. Often, this mild elution process is sufficient to clear enough sites of maternal antibody to allow the Rh typing reaction to occur. The Rh typing can be falsely positive because of the presence of potentiators (e.g., albumin) in commercial Rh typing serum. This is particularly true of the commercial "slide and rapid tube" reagents. A control of the diluent that the company supplied must always be used when typing patients with such reagents. If this control shows a positive result, then the Rh typing should be repeated using a "saline tube" reagent. These reagents can contain small amounts of albumin, so we usually use 10% bovine albumin as a negative control when using such reagents to type patients with positive DAT.[14]

Results in Rh(D) HDN

In HDN associated with anti-D, the results are usually straightforward. The mother is Rh(D) negative with anti-D in her serum. The baby is Rh(D) positive with a positive DAT. Anti-D can be eluted easily from the baby's red cells. If a baby has received enough intrauterine transfusions, the DAT may be negative. The eluate from this blood may or may not be reactive.

Results in HDN Associated with "Other" Antibodies

The most common antibodies, other than anti-D and ABO, to cause HDN are anti-c, anti-E and anti-K. Other antibodies (see Table II) are exceptionally rare causes. The baby's DAT will be positive and the antibodies are usually readily detected in an eluate prepared from the baby's red cells.

If a baby is born with a positive DAT and no antibodies are detected in the mother's serum or the eluate prepared from the baby's red cells, then an antibody to a low frequency antigen should be suspected. The baby's red cells should be tested with monospecific antiglobulin serum (e.g., anti-IgG and anti-complement) to confirm that an IgG antibody is present on the red cells. If the red cells are sensitised with IgG, then one has to explain why the eluate from the baby's red cells and the mother's serum do not react. One answer could be that the baby has inherited a low incidence antigen from the father and the mother has an antibody to this antigen. The reagent red cells used to screen the mother's serum and baby's eluate may lack this antigen. To confirm this, the mother's serum and the eluate from the baby's red cells should be tested against the father's red cells. If a positive reaction is obtained, then a battery of cells containing low incidence antigens will have to be tested to confirm the specificity. Often, the specimens will have to be sent to a reference centre to confirm the specificity.

One unusual alternative explanation for the findings above was reported in 1969 by Clayton et al.[4] At birth, a baby was treated with penicillin. Unfortunately, maternal anti-penicillin had crossed the placenta and reacted with the baby's penicillin-coated red cells, leading to a positive DAT and jaundice. The eluate from the baby's red cells and the mother's serum only reacted with penicillin-coated red cells in vitro.

ABO HDN

The serological findings in ABO HDN are much less helpful in establishing a diagnosis than those found in Rh HDN.

Unlike Rh HDN, there are no reliable tests for the accurate prenatal prediction of ABO HDN. Fortunately, since the disease is usually mild and exchange transfusion is infrequently necessary, early delivery is never indicated.

The disease almost occurs in group A or B infants from group O mothers. This is because A and B individuals rarely make IgG anti-A or anti-B. HDN due to anti-A predominantly affects A_1 infants; that is to say, those who are genetically A_1. Cord blood from A_1 infants with ABO HDN may fail to react with anti-A_1.[13]

Direct Antiglobulin Test: The direct antiglobulin test may be negative even when ABO HDN occurs. If a centrifuge technique is used (rather than a tile method), then less negative results will be observed. Some authors[21,24] have reported that the DAT will be negative more often if performed later than 24 hours after birth. As the clinical symptoms of ABO HDN do not often appear until 24-48 hours after birth, the DAT should be performed on the cord sample that was taken at birth, as well as the later samples. When group A and B babies born of group O mothers have been tested, regardless of their clinical status, DAT results have varied from 14%,[20] when the routine tube (centrifuged) test was used, to 100% of A_1 and B infants when an autoanalyser was used.[10] If one wishes to obtain accurate results when performing manual DAT on babies with possible ABO HDN, it is necessary to check the results microscopically, as sometimes the agglutinisation is not readily visible macroscopically.[21] Some authors,[5,6] and my own findings would agree with this, find that the majority of infants who have clinically and haematologically clear ABO HDN, regularly have a positive DAT.

It has always puzzled everyone why the DAT associated with fetal/maternal ABO incompatibility is often negative. The DAT in Rh HDN is always strongly positive, yet there are only 10–30,000 Rh(D) sites on each red cell, as compared with approximately 250,000 A sites on each red cell from cord blood. One only needs 200/500 IgG molecules per red cell to obtain a positive DAT.[13,14] The anti-A or B eluted from infants' red cells, or the anti-A or B present in their plasma, will readily sensitise adult A or B red cells in vitro to give positive indirect antiglobulin tests.

One obvious difference between the two is that Rh antigens are only present on red cells, whereas ABO antigens are widely distributed in the tissues and body fluids of the infant. Thus although there may be similar amounts of IgG antibody crossing the placenta, comparatively less ABO IgG antibodies may be left to react with red cells. Nevertheless, this is not the complete answer as there is usually free IgG anti-A and/or anti-B present in the infant's plasma, thus it is still surprising that the red cells do not appear to take up enough remaining antibody to yield a positive DAT.

Romano et al[18] showed that the amount of antibody present on red cells from 10 of 15 infants with relatively severe ABO HDN was less than 0.6 µg/ml (220 molecules per red cell). There is some evidence that IgG anti-A is more effective than IgG anti-Rh in bringing about red cell destruction as infant with 0.5 µg anti-A per ml red cells may have a moderately severe haemolytic anaemia, whereas infants with a similar amount of IgG anti-D on their red cells do not.[13]

Recently, Romans et al[19] demonstrated that monogamous bivalency with anti-A and anti-B is necessary to maintain a positive DAT. That is to say, the IgG molecule has to attach to two adjacent A sites with each Fab portion of a single anti-A molecule. On adult red cells there are approximately one million A or B antigenic sites, and they are approximately 85 Å - 100 Å apart. Furthermore, the A and B oligosaccharide chains are multibranched, long flexible structures whose multivalency easily satisfies the two antigen binding sites of a single antibody molecule. In contrast, there are only about 25% of the number of A sites on fetal red cells, and there is a marked deficiency of branched oligosaccharide structures. This could virtually exclude a single anti-A or -B molecule attaching to the red cell by both its Fab portions. Romans et al[19] suggested that if the anti-A or -B are attached by only one Fab portion then the molecules may have a very low affinity and may well come off during the washing process of the DAT. Thus, the DAT would clearly under-estimate the in vivo sensitisation, and hence the risk of red cell destruction of the infant's red cells.

The strong reactions obtained when eluates from infant's red cells with negative DAT are incubated with adult A cells in vitro can be explained by a concentration effect. Not only are there many more antigenic sites on adult red cells, but the proportion of antibody to antigen is greatly increased when two drops of eluate are incubated with one drop of only 2-5% adult red cells.

Eluates Prepared from Baby's Red Cells: One of the most reliable ways to help confirm a diagnosis of ABO HDN is to prepare an eulate from the baby's red cells and then test this eluate, by indirect antiglobulin test, against adult A_1 or B cells. It has been my experience and the experience of others[5,6,26] that this test is almost always positive when ABO HDN occurs. A reactive eluate is usually obtained even when the direct antiglobulin test is negative.

Baby's and Mother's Serum: For ABO HDN to occur, the mother's serum must contain IgG anti-A or anti-B. The baby's serum almost always contains IgG with anti-A and/or anti-B. IgG anti-A and/or anti-B can be demonstrated in the mother's serum by adding 2-ME or DTT to the serum and testing this against adult A_1 or B red cells. The 2-ME or DTT will destroy the activity or IgM antibodies but not affect the reaction of IgG anti-A or anti-B. IgG anti-A or anti-B can directly agglutinate adult A or B red cells, or may only be detected by the indirect antiglobulin test. Haemolysins present in the mother's serum may be IgM or IgG.

Rh(D) IMMUNE GLOBULIN (Rh IG)

Candidates for Rh IG are mothers who are Rh (D) and D^u negative; have no detectable anti-D; and, deliver a D or D^u positive baby. Rh negative mothers who abort, have amniocentesis, antepartum haemorrhage or ectopic pregnancy, are often considered as candidates.

If the newborn is known to be Rh(D) positive and the bloodbank receives a request for Rh IG, the following procedures should be performed before administering Rh IG to the mother:

1. Obtain a new blood sample from the mother to investigate fetomaternal haemorrhage.
2. ABO group mother (to identify sample).
3. Rh(D) type mother (including a microscopic D^u test).
4. Test mother's serum for unexpected antibodies.

5. Some workers perform a compatibility test between the mother's red cells and the sample of diluted Rh IG, but I do not feel this is necessary.

Detection of Fetal Red Cells: Approximately 1-2% of women who receive Rh IG post-delivery develop Rh antibodies prior to or during a subsequent Rh positive pregnancy. These "failures" include: (1) those women who, although they have no detectable antibody at delivery, are already immunized; and, (2) those women who have more than 15 ml of fetal red cells in their circulation. The incidence of fetomaternal haemorrhage (FMH) of this size is 0.3%.[25] Immunisation in this latter group can often be prevented if the FMH is identified and a larger than standard dose of Rh IG administered.

Serological clues that an FMH of more than 30 ml of whole blood has occurred are:

1. A mother who was typed as Rh(D) negative (D^u negative) on her initial visit, types as D^u positive post partum (i.e., weak mixed field reaction with anti-D by indirect antiglobulin test).
2. Rh immune globulin crossmatch incompatible.

The D^u test, if performed efficiently, (i.e., read microscopically) is the best practical screening test available.[1,16] Agglutination in the microscope phase of the D^u test may not indicate a massive fetomaternal haemorrhage, but may be caused by:

1. The patient being a weak D^u.
2. The reagent anti-D "slide and rapid tube" test serum not being standardized for close microscopic reading in the antiglobulin test.
3. Contamination of the anti-D reagent with another weaker antibody that reacts with the patient's red cells.

The results of the D^u test can be confirmed by the acid-elution procedure (e.g., Kleihauer-Betke test) for detection of fetal red cells. Table V shows some uses of the Kleihauer-Betke method.

Quantitation of Fetal Red Cells The number of fetal red cells present is usually expressed as a proportion of adult red cells in the same sample. It is important that the following factors are taken into account:[13]

a) Fetal red cells are larger than adult cells, so that the volume present will be greater than that indicated by the number present.

b) Not all fetal red cells stain darkly by the acid-elution method.

c) An arbitrary figure for maternal red cell volume has to be assumed.

TABLE V

SOME USES OF THE KLEIHAUER-BETKE METHOD

1. Screening for and quantitating FMH
2. Determining origin of red cells in amniotic fluid
3. Monitoring effectiveness of intrauterine transfusions
4. Measuring survival of red cells with HbF
5. Identifying mislabelled samples (eg, mother/baby samples)

Making the following assumptions that: a) fetal red cells have a volume about 22% larger than adult cells; b) that about 92% of fetal cells stain darkly; c) that the average red cell volume of a recently delivered woman is 1800 ml; the absolute volume of fetal red cells present can be estimated by the following formula:[13]

$$\text{FMH (ml)} = \frac{2400}{\text{no. of adult RBC: no. of fetal RBC}}$$

or:

% fetal red cells X 50.

COMPATIBILITY TESTING FOR EXCHANGE TRANSFUSIONS

Donor blood selected for exchange transfusions should: 1) lack the red cell antigens corresponding to the maternal antibodies; 2) be crossmatched with the mother's serum; and, 3) be less than three days old. The donor blood should, of course, have been screened for unexpected antibodies, hepatitis and syphilis.

For ABO HDN, group O red cells of the same Rh type as the baby should be used. In order to avoid transfusing more anti-A and anti-B, either packed, partially packed, or frozen deglycerolised blood can be used. Some workers prefer to suspend red cells in compatible plasma (e.g., group AB).

In Rh(D) and "other" HDN, blood of the baby's own ABO group is usually used when the mother's serum is ABO-compatible. If the mother's serum is ABO-incompatible with the baby's group, then group O blood lacking the appropriate antigen (e.g., Rh negative, if Rh HDN) is usually transfused, using the same criteria as previously discussed. Table VI illustrates the choices of blood for exchange transfusions.

TABLE VI

BLOOD FOR EXCHANGE TRANSFUSION FOR Rh HDN

(Rh - Compatible with Mother's Serum)

	Mother's ABO			
Baby's ABO	O	A	B	AB
O	O	O	O	
A	A or O	A	A or O	A or O
B	B or O	B or O	B	B or O
AB		AB or A	AB or B	AB, A or B

As discussed previously, I would recommend crossmatching only at 37 C. I would incubate equal volumes of a 2% suspension of red donor cells in LISS with maternal serum (or baby's serum or eluate made into LISS) at 37 C for 10-15 mins. and then following centrifugation; wash four times and add antiglobulin serum.

The mother's serum is used for the compatibility testing since the offending antibody is present in greater amounts than in the baby's serum. If the mother's serum is unavailable, then baby's serum, or an eluate prepared from the baby's red cells should be used. In repeated exchange transfusions, units of the same blood type should be used. Some workers recommend crossmatching these subsequent units with the baby's serum, in addition to the mother's serum, in case there is intradonor incompatibility from any antibodies in donor units used for the previous transfusions.

IgG SUBCLASS AND HDN

There is evidence that IgG1 and Rh antibodies are produced more often than

IgG3 Rh antibodies in pregnant women. There is also data to suggest that if they are G1m(a) positive, they will be more likely to make antibodies carrying G1m(a), as opposed to G1m(f).[22]

There is some evidence to suggest that IgG1 is preferentially transported across the placenta.[22] IgG3 antibodies are known to be generally more efficient at causing immune red cell destruction,[7,14] but little is known about the differences in HDN.

Since IgG1 antibodies cross the placenta first, fetal red cells should have longer exposure to antibody. In contrast, IgG3 antibodies may not ever achieve maternal levels due to their late transfer-across the placenta. Schanfield and co-workers[22] recently showed that infants from mothers with IgG1 antibodies had low mean cord haemoglobin levels and higher mean cord bilirubin levels with lower postnatal rise-bilirubin. They suggest this reflects a longer period of chronic red cell destruction due to the lower haemolytic potential of IgG1 antibodies when the amount of antibody is not replenished. In contrast, infants from mothers with IgG3 antibodies had a higher mean haemoglobin and lower mean cord bilirubin; however, they had significantly higher postnatal rise in bilirubin (Table VII).

TABLE VII

RELATIONSHIP OF IgG SUBCLASS TO INDICATORS OF SEVERITY OF HDN

	Cord		Postnatal Rise in Bilirubin
Subclass	Haemoglobin	Bilirubin	mg/dl/hour
IgGI	9.87 (n = 4)	8.80 (n = 5)	0.24 (n = 2)
IgG3	13.90 (n = 3)	3.67 (n = 3)	0.52 (n = 4)
IgGl + 3	12.7 (n = 3)	3.73 (n = 3)	0.25 (n = 2)

Schanfield et al[22] have also suggested that within the IgG1 subclass, G1m(a) antibodies may be significantly less haemolytic than G1m(f). They found that mothers of moderately and severely affected infants showed a striking absence of G1m(a) positive IgG1 Rh antibodies. The majority were

G1m(f), G3m(b), G3m(g) or mixtures of IgG1 and IgG3. In addition, there was an overall under representation of the phenotype Gm(f, 3, a, b, g) which should occur in 50% of the cases; amongst those that did occur, the majority of the antibodies were G1m(a).

It was suggested that the differences in transport of subclass-specific antibody across the placenta and their haemolytic potential, may account for some of the discrepancies noted between maternal antibody titres and severity of HDN. For example, a mother with an Rh antibody, titre 2048, which is all IgG3 may deliver a not too severely affected infant. However, the child would probably need therapy postnatally. In contrast, an IgG1, Glm(f) antibody, of similar titre, may cause severe HDN in utero leading to a stillborn fetus. An Rh IgG1 antibody of lower titre (e.g., 64-128) might be associated with a mildly affected infant at birth, requiring no further treatment; while, an IgG3 antibody of the same titre might be associated with an infant mildly affected at birth but subsequently becoming severely affected.

In summary, IgG1 antibodies appear to cause greater destruction in utero, followed by a more benign postnatal course. In contrast, IgG3 antibodies appear to cause less destruction in utero, but are associated with a much more severe course postnatally.

REFERENCES

1. American Association of Blood Banks: Technical Manual, ed 7, Washington DC, American Association of Blood Banks, 1977.

2. Bowman, J.M.: Suppression of Rh isoimmunization, Obstet. and Gynec. 52:385, 1978.

3. Browdy, S: Should every newborn infant be given a Coombs test? Clin. Pediat. 10:427, 1971.

4. Clayton, E,M., Hyun, B.H., Palumbo, V.N. et al: Penicillin-induced positive Coombs test in a newborn. Am.J.Clin.Path. 52:370, 1969.

5. Desjardins, L., Chintu, C. and A. Zipursky: The spectrum of ABO haemolytic disease of the newborn infant. J.Pediat. 95:447, 1979.

6. Dufour, D.R. and W.P. Monoghan: ABO haemolytic disease of the newborn. Am.J.Clin.Path. 3:369, 1980

7. Engelfriet, C.P., Von dem Bourne, A.E.G., Beckers, D. et al: Autoimmune haemolytic anaemia: Serological and immunochemical characteristics of the autoantibodies; mechanisms of cell destruction. Series Haematologica VII:328, 1974.

8. Fitzsimmons J.M. and P.A. Morel: The effects of red blood cell suspending media on haemagglutination and the antiglobulin test. Transfusion 19:81, 1979.

9. Giblett E.R.: Blood group alloantibodies: an assessment of some laboratory practices. Transfusion 17:299, 1977.

10. Hsu, T.C.S., Rosenfield, R.E. and P. Rubinstein: Instrumented PVP-augmented antiglobulin tests. III. IgG-coated cells in ABO incompatible babies; depressed haemoglobin levels in type A babies of type O mothers. Vox Sang 26:326, 1974.

11. Issitt, P.D.: Antibodies Reactive at 30 Centigrade, Room Temperature and Below. In: Clinically Significant and Insignificant Antibodies, Washington DC, American Association of Blood Banks, 1979, p. 13.

12. Kline, W.E.: Chemistry of Blood Group Antigens and Antibodies in Haemolytic Disease of the Newborn. In: A Seminar on Perinatal Blood Banking. Washington DC, American Association of Blood Banks, 1978, p.1.

13. Mollison, P.L.: Blood Transfusion in Clinical Medicine, ed. 5, Oxford, Blackwell Scientific Publications, 1972.

14. Petz, L.D. and G. Garratty: Acquired Immune Haemolytic Anaemias, New York, Churchill Livingstone, 1980.

15. Polesky, H.: Blood group antibodies in prenatal sera - results of screening 43,000 individuals. Minnesota Med. 50:602, 1967.

16. Polesky, H.F. and E.S. Sebring: Detection of fetal maternal haemorrhage: an evaluation of serological tests related to Rh_o(D) immune globulin (human). Transfusion 11:162, 1971.

17. Pollack, W., Ascari, W.Q., Crispen, J.F., O'Connor, R.R., and T.Y. Ho: Studies on Rh prophylaxis. II. Rh immune prophylaxis after transfusion with Rh-positive blood. Transfusion 11:340, 1971.

18. Romano, E.L., Hughes-Jones, N.C., and P.L. Mollison: Direct antiglobulin reaction in ABO-haemolytic disease of the newborn. Br. Med. J. 1:524, 1973.

19. Romans, D.G., Tilley, C.A. and K.J. Dorrington: Monogamous bivalency of IgG antibodies. I. Deficiency of branched ABHI-active oligosaccharide chains on red cells of infants causes the weak antiglobulin reactions in haemolytic disease of the newborn due to ABO incompatibility. J. Immunol. 124:2807, 1980.

20. Rosenfield, R.E. and G. Ohno: A-B haemolytic disease of the newborn. Rev. Haemat. 10:231, 1955.

21. Sabo, B.H.: Evaluation of the Neonatal Direct Antiglobulin Test: Notes on Low-Frequency Antigens in Haemolytic Disease of the Newborn. In: A Seminar on Perinatal Blood Banking, Washington DC, American Association of Blood Banks, 1978, p.31.

22. Schanfield, M.S.: Human Immunoglobulin (IgG) Subclasses and their Biological Properties. In: Blood Bank Immunology, Washington DC, American Association of Blood Banks, 1977, p.97.

23. Spielmann, W. and S. Seidl: Prevalence of irregular red cell antibodies and their significance in blood transfusion and antenatal care. Vox. Sang. 26:551, 1974.

24. Walker, R.H.: ABO-Haemolytic Disease of the Newborn. In: Walker, R.H. (ed), Haemolytic Disease of the Newborn, Chicago, 1971, p.99.

25. World Health Organisation Technical Report Series No. 468: Prevention of Rh sensitisation. Report of a WHO Scientific Group, Geneva, 1971.

26. Yunis, E. and R. Bridges: The serologic diagnosis of ABO-haemolytic disease of the newborn. Am.J.Clin.Path. 41:1, 1964.

----

2. THE LABORATORY INVESTIGATION OF ABO HAEMOLYTIC DISEASE OF THE NEWBORN AND DANGERS ARISING FROM THE TRANSFUSION OF GROUP O DONOR-BLOOD CONTAINING AB BLOODGROUP SUBSTANCE OF ANIMAL ORIGIN

J.W. LOCKYER

Since the year 1923 when Ottenburg[3] advanced his idea that iso-antibodies might occasionally cross the placenta and be the cause of neonatal jaundice a steady and continuous flow of scientific and technical data has been published about such antibodies and their role in ABO haemolytic disease of the newborn (ABO HDN). As a result of this it can be said that there are few branches of bloodgroup serology which have had more written about them. Gold and Butler[2] in their monograph of ABO haemolytic disease of the newborn give no fewer than 670 references to published work associated with this disease. In spite of this vast amount of information there are many complex problems still unsolved and requiring further investigation. Among these are:

1) the frequent lack of a positive direct anti-human globulin test on the cord cells of infants suffering from ABO HDN
2) the nature of antibodies causing ABO HDN
3) the specificity of the cross-reacting antibody
4) the structure and configuration of the combining site of the pathogenic anti-A, anti-B and of their corresponding AB antigens
5) the chemistry of these antigens in the red cell membrane.

It is unfortunate that with so many antenatal tests available for examining maternal sera aimed at screening out those capable of bringing about ABO HDN, and with as many also available for examining the cord cells with an aim to confirming diagnosis, the haematologist is not able to provide the obstetrician or paediatrician with the same valuable help in predicting possible severity of the disease as he is able to give following the normal antenatal laboratory investigation for rhesus incompatibility.

As a result of the vast amount of research carried out on group O sera taken from cases of ABO HDN the following antibodies appear to be associated, though not necessarily directly involved in the disease process:

Anti-C (Wiener)
IgM Anti-A-B 'naturally' occurring
IgM anti-A-B immune
IgG anti-A-B
Anti-A-B haemolysins
Cross-reacting anti-A/B symmetrical
Cross-reacting anti-A/B asymmetrical
IgM anti-A^{P}
IgG anti-A^{P}.

A large amount of research into the importance of these different antibodies has recently been carried out at the South-West Regional Blood Transfusion Laboratories, Bristol, England and has formed part of a thesis on this subject by the author of this paper. From the results obtained it would appear that most, if not all of the maternal antibodies are associated in bringing about some destruction of the fetal ABO incompatible red cells though some are obviously much more important than others, and it is possible that insufficient attention has been given in the past to such antibodies as the cross-reacting forms of alpha-beta particularly those of the asymmetric variety.

Symmetric and asymmetric CRA are classified by their reaction when tested against A_1 and B cells after having been previously eluted from either A_1 or B cells. Eluates prepared from A_1 cells incubated with heat inactivated group O immune - serum will, when titrated against A_1 and B cells by saline agglutination technique show either symmetric cross-reacting activity, that is, it will have equal potency against both the A_1 and B cells, or it will have asymmetric activity in which case the cross-reacting antibody will have a much greater activity against A_1 than B or against B rather than A.

By looking closely at the stimulating effect of different forms of human and animal A antigens on group O mothers, one can show that whereas vaccine prophylaxis and bacterial infection produce mainly symmetric CRA, human A and B antigen produce the asymmetric form. Where A is the stimulating antigen the antibody specificity will be CR ( ), and where B is the antigen the antibody specificity will be CR( ) . From the work carried out the asymmetric type of the CRA appears to be the major antibody involved in ABO HDN, and that such antibody is produced from a fetal/maternal leak of plasma or red cell antigens rather than vaccine prophylaxis or bacterial infection.

It would therefore seem reasonable to suggest that the asymmetric type of cross-reacting anti-A-B is one of the antibodies to investigate during the antenatal period.

Cord blood studies have shown that both the A-B antigen site density levels of the fetal red cells and the amount of free A or B antigen in the plasma seriously affect the degree of severity of red cell destruction. In affected cases the appropriate number of A sites per cord cell is in the region of 290,000 to 810,000. The unaffected infant's cells lie between 120,000 and 240,000. Experiments have shown that both red cell and plasma A and B antigens are in a constant state of competition for the chance to combine with the maternal placenta-crossing antibody. The presence of strong cell antigens and weak plasma antigens would almost certainly result in a severely affected infant, whereas a high titre antibody in the presence of strong plasma antigen could result in an unaffected infant. This might well be one of the major reasons why when testing the maternal antenatal serum for high titre anti-A-B and finding a high titre it does not necessarily follow that the infant will be affected.

From the experimental work carried out it would appear that the antenatal assessment of severity of ABO HDN can never be made with the same degree of accuracy as can rhesus, as a number of parameters are involved which cannot be measured antenatally, such as fetal A-B antigen strength and the amount of free A-B substance in the fetal plasma.

From the investigations carried out it would appear that four major factors control how severely an infant which is ABO incompatible with its mother will be affected by the disease. Firstly there is the type specificity and strength of maternal antibody (probably IgG - and/or cross-reacting asymmetric -). Secondly, the A or B antigen site density on the fetal red cells. Thirdly, the amount of free A or B soluble antigen in the infant's plasma. Finally, an early leak of A or B antigen from the fetus into the mother.

When preparing blood for exchange transfusion in ABO haemolytic disease of the newborn several methods of preparation are available. Within this laboratory blood is used from group O donors, tested and found to be free of both alpha beta haemolysins and high titre alpha beta agglutinins. Such bloods should therefore be totally compatible with infant's red cells and should not complicate the haemolytic process. Blood used in this way should be more than 24 hours old to avoid the transmission of cytomegalovirus and less than 3 days old to reduce increased risk of potassium toxicity. Approximately two-thirds of the plasma should be removed to compensate for the higher fetal haemoglobin levels. As an alternative to this method, washed group O cells suspended in inert AB serum can be used equally well.

The dangers of adding AB blood group specific substance of animal origin (Witebsky substance) to human group O blood prior to exchange transfusion cannot be over-emphasised. The practice is both outdated and totally unnecessary.

In adult transfusion the introduction of biological material of animal origin can create an immune response against it within the recipient which might later give rise to difficulties should a recipient receive injections or vaccination material obtained from the same animal species. It must be remembered that purified blood group specific substance only neutralises the IgM alpha-beta agglutinins and has little or no inhibitory effect upon any IgG alpha-beta antibodies which might be present. Under normal circumstances, in a transfusion of group O blood containing low-titre alpha-beta agglutinins to group A-B or AB recipients most, if not all the agglutinins will be neutralised by the recipient's free A-B substance in its plasma. The presence of any IgG alpha-beta antibodies in donor plasma is therefore the more dangerous and will be more likely to bring about ABO incompatibility. A further complication can arise in that any excess A-B substance left free will cause a marked post-transfusion increase in the recipient's IgM anti-A-B titre and the development of potent IgG anti-A-B. Whilst these must not be considered too great a complication when transfusing male patients, the stimulation of such antibodies in group O females of child bearing age could have a much more serious affect, particularly in those cases where the person later becomes involved in an ABO incompatible pregnancy.

When exchange transfusing babies affected with ABO haemolytic disease of the newborn, the practice of using group O blood neutralised with animal group specific substance can give rise to increased rather than decreased destruction of the baby's red cells: this can occur if the group O donor blood contains IgG anti-A-B in addition to the IgM. These IgG antibodies will not be neutralised by the A-B substance and will increase the quantity of free incompatible IgG antibody available for reacting with the infant's red cell, thereby increasing the haemolytic state. The danger of transfusing immune complex is also a reality.

In modern clinical bloodtransfusion practice there is no need for adding potentially dangerous animal A-B substance which is manufactured solely as a laboratory reagent and, as clearly stated by the American Federal Drug Administration Committee[1], should not be used intravenously.

REFERENCES

1. Code of Federal Regulations, Chapter 21, Washington DC, 1980, p.162.
2. Gold, E.R. and N.R. Butler: ABO Haemolytic Disease of the Newborn, J. Wright & Son Ltd., Bristol, 1972.
3. Ottenburg, R.: The Aetiology of Eclampsia. J.Amer.med.Assoc. 81:295 1923.

3. HAEMOLYTIC DISEASE: CLINICAL DIAGNOSIS

M.M. KERR

In a well ordered society, with every woman wanting, and receiving, impeccable prenatal care, with no mislaid laboratory reports, with complete rhesus genotyping, and with all cord blood specimens taken properly and despatched promptly to the laboratory with a 24 hour, 7 day a week service, it is rarely necessary to make a clinical diagnosis of rhesus incompatibility, unless perhaps to assess the severity of the process in individual infants. Clinicians can merely sit back and await the telephoned results from their colleagues in the laboratory.

We do not, alas, live and work in such a perfect world and I shall therefore pretend that I, as a clinician have no forewarning of a potential case. I need therefore, to be fully alert, as always when examining any new baby, and to use my eyes and my hands. Despite pretending that I have been given no warning, for the sake of clarity I shall divide the clinical picture of affected babies into the three conventional groups, although we all of us know that there can be no sharp dividing line.

TABLE I

THE CLASSIC CASE
(Icterus Gravis)

Pallor $\pm$	
Jaundice - early onset	
Yellow staining of:	cord
	parts of body
	whole baby
	gastric aspirate

In the classic case of icterus gravis (Table I) the baby may, or may not be pale, this obviously depending on the haemoglobin level. He will become obviously jaundiced, possibly by the age of 15 minutes after birth, and certainly within the first 24 hours. He may look jaundiced at birth because there may be staining of some or all parts of his body due to his immersion in golden liquor amnii.

When we examine him we will find a varying degree of hepatosplenomegaly. There may well be scattered petechiae and there may or may not be some oedema. This may be partly related to his gestational age rather than to the severity of the haemolytic process.

TABLE II

THE SEVERE CASE

(Hydrops Fetalis)

Generalised oedema

Pallor

Cyanosis $\pm$

Massive hepatosplenomegaly

Generalised petechiae

In the severe case (Table II) - hydrops fetalis - there will be gross generalised oedema, pallor and possibly cyanosis. The hepatosplenomegaly will be massive and there will be generalised petechiae. The abdomen will be distended, partly due to the hepatosplenomegaly and partly to ascites. Pleural effusions may be present. These, plus the low haemoglobin and the abdominal distension, will certainly have caused problems in initiating and maintaining respiration.

In the mild case, sometimes called congenital haemolytic anaemia, there may or may not be obvious pallor, jaundice may never occur - at least not until after the age of 24 hours, and there may or may not be any enlargement of liver or spleen. These are the babies who slowly become anaemic due to continuing mild haemolysis - this may not be obvious until the pallor is investigated when they are several weeks old (Table III).

TABLE III

THE MILD CASE

(Congenital Haemolytic Anaemia)

Pallor ±

Mild jaundice ± - late onset

Hepatosplenomegaly ±

Late anaemia

I have described many clinical findings - but with almost everyone there may be another explanation. We must therefore now look at the differential diagnosis. With a hydropic infant we really only have to consider the homozygous form of alpha-thalassaemia - usually stillborn, always fatal - and that strange rare condition of polyserositis where we find massive ascites and pleural effusions of completely unknown aetiology.

Now let us consider the infant who presents with obvious pallor at birth. There may have been fetal bleeding

- feto-maternal
- feto-placental

or from a ruptured vasa praevia.

With multiple pregnancy we must consider the twin-twin transfusion syndrome. If delivery was by caesarian section, was the placenta anterior and therefore incised before the baby could be delivered, with inevitably some loss of fetal blood? Then we must remember the occasional accident. Sadly we have had a fatal case where a fetal vessel was punctured by the insertion of an intra-uterine monitoring catheter. Remember too, the extreme pallor of severe birth asphyxia - the old name after all was asphyxia pallida. Pallor noticeable within a few hours of birth may be the presenting sign in severe cyanotic congenital heart disease, and also in overwhelming septicaemia.

Let us now turn to early jaundice (Table IV). Here we must think of, and exclude, ABO and other incompatibilities such as Kell and Duffy. Remember too the possibility of pyknocytosis and spherocytosis. Severe viral and protozoal infections acquired in utero will result in early jaundice as will toxic substances, such as naptha, taken by or given to the mother.

TABLE IV

Differential Diagnosis

EARLY JAUNDICE

ABO Incompatibility
Other incompatibilities - Kell, Duffy, etc.
Spherocytosis
Pyknocytosis
Severe intrauterine infections -- viral
protozoal
Toxic substances

Logically, we must now consider possible reasons for jaundice appearing rather later (Table V). To the causes just mentioned we must add glucuronyl transferase deficiency in preterm infants, glucose-6-phosphate dehydrogenase deficiency, the mild form of alphathalassaemia, postnatal infections (mostly bacterial), and a great list of other causes.

TABLE V

Differential Diagnosis

LATER JAUNDICE

As before
+
G-6PD deficiency
Glucuronyl transferase deficiency in the preterm
Alphathalassaemia (mild form)
Infection
Etcetera
Etcetera

Enlargement of liver and spleen will of course be found in ABO and other incompatibilities, in spherocytosis, and associated with intrauterine infections (Table VI).

TABLE VI

Differential Diagnosis
HEPATOSPLENOMEGALY

ABO incompatibility
Other incompatibilities
Spherocytosis
Severe intrauterine infections
Toxic substances

Petechiae are not all that uncommon in the newborn (Table VII). When associated with thrombocytopenia we must consider again viral and protozoal infections, we must think of maternal ideopathic thrombocytopenic purpura and of autoimmune thrombocytopenia. With a normal platelet count, we must consider trauma (particularly in large babies), haemorrhagic disease of the newborn (although skin manifestations are rare) and, as an extreme rarity, congenital leukemia.

TABLE VII

Differential Diagnosis
PETECHIAE

Other causes of thrombocytopenia :-
- viral and protozoal infections
- maternal ITP
- autoimmune

Trauma
Haemorrhagic disease of the newborn
Congenital leukemia

Lastly, our differential diagnosis in the very mild case (Table VIII). There may have been a small fetal bleed from one of the causes already referred to. There may have been internal haemorrhage in the baby - to brain, beneath the liver capsule or to the gut. Aplastic anaemia is excessively rare, but has to be kept in mind. Finally, in this era of intensive care, with frequent measurements of acid base, electrolytes, drug levels,and a whole battery of other tests never let us forget that we, the clinicians, may have caused the mild anaemia quite simply by the amount of blood we have removed from our small patient.

TABLE VIII

THE MILD CASE
(Congenital Haemolytic Anaemia)
Differential Diagnosis

Fetal bleeding -- as before
Occult postnatal haemorrhage
Aplastic anaemia
Iatrogenic

I have reminded you that the clinical diagnosis of Rhesus incompatibility is not always simple. How very dependent therefore are we clinicians on our colleagues in the laboratory.

----

4. DISCUSSION

Moderator: J.O. FORFAR

J.G. JOLLY (Chandigahr, India): The positivity of direct Coombs, reported recently, has certainly shaken a number of workers. I should like to be enlightened as to the possible explanation and to hear the experiences of other workers. Ever since this report came out, we have tried to be more careful with the direct Coombs test, as well as looking at the various types of sera which we were getting, but somehow we have not been able to get the results that were quoted earlier.

Secondly, in addition to Rh, ABO and other causes of neonatal jaundice, we too have tried to investigate physiological jaundice and, surprisingly, a sizable number of cases have been found to be G-6-PD deficient. Of 1,377 cases investigated G-6-PD was the dominant cause in 38%. Rh incompatibility was next with 14%; prematurity, 11%; ABO, 9% and unclassified, 32%. When we looked at this record and the therapy that was required, we came to the conclusion that those with Rh incompatibility needed a higher percentage of exchange transfusions or more than one exchange transfusion, which perhaps was directly related to the severity of the disease. However, although the frequency of G-6-PD deficiency was highest the percentage of those requiring an exchange was lowest when compared with Rh and ABO. In fact, a large proportion of this group did not require any active treatment. It would therefore be appropriate to conclude that a sizable percentage of cases previously labelled as physiological jaundice were in fact due to G-6-PD deficiency. This appears to be the situation in India where we have about a 7% G-6-PD deficiency in the normal population. I have examined some 15,000 normal healthy donors and it ranged from 7% to 9%. It may be variable, but perhaps this is an important cause, and a sizable number of cases which are not severe and which are left on the pretext that this is possibly physiological jaundice might need further investigation.

C.A. HOLMAN (London, U.K.): I should like to support Mr. Garratty in his comments about LISS but I would offer a warning. At a workshop held in London earlier in 1980 it was made quite clear that many homemade LISS reagents and some of the commercial LISS reagents were quite unsatisfactory. A very strict quality control has to be maintained and as it takes a fair amount of expensive apparatus to do it it should be limited in its production. It certainly picks up antibodies that we are not picking up by other methods and it creates a certain amount of confusion in the obstetricians. We keep finding, for example, anti-E naturally occurring antibody - which we have not seen before.

Mr Garratty made the point that a lot of trouble might be saved by not reporting or finding these naturally occurring antibodies, but in our experience it is very important both to find them and to report them. For example,if - as we do - a clinician has a large number of Le(a- b-) patients he can be confronted at delivery with the need for blood for them which it is difficult to provide, whereas if it was known in advance that they had the antibodies the blood could be available and there would be no last-minute crossmatching problems. I should also like to point out that if these naturally occurring antibodies should be missed and not followed up, then from time to time there will be a case of haemolytic disease due to a conversion in that particular mother from naturally occurring to immune antibody. I myself have seen a girl who was listed as naturally occurring anti-MIA and VW who subsequently produced an immune anti-VW - her husband being VW positive -with most severe haemolytic disease requiring infusion and transfusion.

W.H. OUWEHAND (Amsterdam, Netherlands): In our laboratories we have done a few hundred serologies on haemolytic disease of the newborn and we could not correlate the severity of the haemolysis with the subclasses that we could show on the red cell surfaces of the newborn. We have seen in autoimmune haemolytic anaemia that subclasses are of great importance, but that cannot be said of haemolytic disease of the newborn. Quantifying the antibody may well give us more insight into red cell destruction in the newborn.

R.L. McSHINE (Groningen, Netherlands): Considering the strength of the direct antiglobulin tests in haemolytic disease of the newborn, could this be dependent on a subclass of IgG anti-A on the infant's red cells and on the quality and the composition of the anti-IgG serum which is used?

G. GARRATTY (Los Angeles, U.S.): I do not think so, but I would bow to anybody from Amsterdam on this. They have a lot more experience than I do of subclasses. As far as I know, commercial anti-IgG does not have any subclass specificity. There will be no variation in the anti-IgG 1, 2, 3 and 4. A different determinant - a more general IgG determinant - is reacting.

THE SUPPLY OF ANTI-RHESUS (D) IMMUNOGLOBULIN IN THE NETHERLANDS

E.E. REERINK-BRONGERS

1964 was an important year in the history of haemolytic disease of the newborn. It was then that Clarke in England and Freda in the U.S. published, almost simultaneously, that rhesus (D) immunisation due to pregnancy could be prevented by administering immunoglobulin preparations containing a high titre of anti-rhesus (D) antibodies to the mother. This was the beginning of the end of the battle against this disease, first described in 1892 by Ballantyne,and whose pathogenesis was exposed in 1941 by Levine.

In the Netherlands, a working party consisting of Dr. E. Borst-Eilers, Dr. Chr. van der Weerdt, Professor Dr. G.J. Kloosterman and Dr. C. Dudok de Wit started a campaign for the prevention of rhesus (D) haemolytic disease in 1964. In 1965, the first batch of anti-rhesus (D) immunoglobulin was produced by Dr. H.W. Krijnen at the Central Laboratory of the Bloodtransfusion Service of the Netherlands Red Cross.

This specific immunoglobulin is prepared from plasma containing a high titre of anti-rhesus (D) antibodies in exactly the same way as other immunoglobulin preparations: i.e., by ethanol fractionation at low temperature and at low pH. This results in an immunoglobulin preparation containing 16% protein, mainly IgG, but the other immunoglobulins are also present in small quantities, and traces of other plasma proteins as well. The starting material is plasma containing ca 30 µg anti-rhesus (D) immunoglobulin per ml (haemagglutination titre 1:2000 - 1:4000). In the Netherlands there is a "cohort" of 150 faithful donors who together provide the amount of plasma required. Nine of them are women who have been immunised by pregnancies. The others (107 men and 34 women) have been immunised intentionally, with their consent, by three intravenous injections of 0 R_2r erythrocytes from a donor who has given blood at least ten times without having been involved in cases of post-transfusion hepatitis. This donor is K negative and Fy^a negative. The titre of the anti-rhesus (D) antibodies is maintained by I.V. injections of the same 0 R_2r erythrocytes at intervals of approximately four months. The donors are plasmapheresed 10 - 11 times a year, the yield being 560 ml plasma a time. The interval between plasmaphereses is at least one month.

It is due to these donors that since 1969 anti-rhesus (D) immunoglobulin has been provided at the public expense in doses of 200 µg to rhesus (D) negative women without anti-rhesus (D) antibodies who have given birth to a rhesus (D) positive child. In the beginning, anti-rhesus (D) immunoglobulin was only given after the birth of the first child - provided mother and child were ABO compatible. In 1970, the supply of anti-rhesus (D) immunoglobulin was sufficient to offer it after the birth of a second child as well and irrespective of ABO compatibility. By the end of 1971 there was no further need for restrictions, and anti-rhesus (D) could be provided for all rhesus (D) negative women without anti-rhesus (D) antibodies who had delivered a rhesus (D) positive child.

The result of this policy is shown in Table I. Apparently the number of rhesus (D) immunisations is declining but it has not fallen away to zero. The causes of the persistence of rhesus (D) immunisation might be:

1. anti-rhesus (D) not being given after previous deliveries. This would probably mainly affect immigrant women from Mediterranean countries.
2. Errors in the determination of the rhesus (D) factor either of the baby or of the mother (rare).
3. Rhesus (D) immunisation having already taken place prior to or during a first pregnancy.
4. The given amount of anti-rhesus (D) immunoglobulin being insufficient (fetomaternal transfusions of more than 50 ml).

To lower the incidence of rhesus (D) sensitisation still further anti-rhesus (D) immunoglobulin should also be given to all rhesus (D) negative women without anti-rhesus (D) antibodies:

1. after every abortion (75 µg)
2. after amniocentesis (early amniocentesis 75 µg; late 200 µg)
3. after difficult external versions and other procedures which might cause fetomaternal haemorrhage.

A further measure would be to introduce the Kleihauer test as a routine determination and to adapt the dosage of anti-rhesus (D) immunoglobulin to the extent of the fetomaternal haemorrhage (10 µg per ml fetal blood).

TABLE I

	A	B		C		D
	number of live births	anti-D determinations 8th month		anti-D+ (1st time)		ampoules anti-D 200 µg
		1	2	1	2	
1969	247600	29860	(12%)	1058	(3.5%)	7085
1970	238900	28232	(12%)	811	(2.9%)	10884
1971	227180	27486	(12%)	584	(2.1%)	19654
1972	214133	25661	(12%)	505	(2.0%)	21615
1973	195188	23908	(12%)	324	(1.4%)	18465
1974	185982	23313	(13%)	295	(1.3%)	18543
1975	177876	22559	(13%)	213	(0.9%)	23159
1976	177090	22624	(13%)	137	(0.6%)	23076
1977	173269	22162	(13%)	102	(0.5%)	22550
1978	175550	22440	(13%)	106	(0.5%)	21367
1979	174979	22425	(13%)	?		22033

A number of live births per year in the Netherlands

B 1 - number of anti-rhesus(D) determinations in 8th month of pregnancy performed by the Central Laboratory of the Bloodtransfusion Service of the Netherlands Red Cross**

2 - number of anti-rhesus(D) determinations expressed as percentage of the number of live births

C 1 - number of first-time positive results of anti(D) determinations from column B

2 - number of these positive results expressed as percentage of number of anti(D) determinations

D number of ampoules anti-rhesus(D) immunoglobulin @ 200 µg provided at public expense in the Netherlands

**(Some 75% of all determinations in the Netherlands are done in Amsterdam: the other 25% in Groningen at the Institute for Bloodgroup Serology)

To prevent sensitisation during pregnancies, antenatal administration of anti-rhesus (D) immunoglobulin in the 28th and 34th week is recommended. This, however, would require more than three times the amount of anti-rhesus (D) immunoglobulin now used and would be prohibitively costly in terms of any gain, as well as involving immunising three times as many donors.

----

2. ANTI-RHESUS (D) IMMUNOGLOBULIN: INDICATIONS, CLINICAL USE AND EFFECT ON INCIDENCE OF HAEMOLYTIC DISEASE OF THE NEWBORN

J. BENNEBROEK GRAVENHORST

INTRODUCTION

It is a well established fact that Rh (D) antibodies develop in Rh (D) negative subjects who receive Rh positive erythrocytes. The major cause of Rh immunisation is pregnancy in a Rh negative woman carrying a Rh positive fetus. Although in principle, the circulations of mother and child are completely separate, small volumes of fetal erythrocytes may enter the maternal circulation during labour and delivery. Some Rh negative individuals respond with the formation of Rh (D) antibodies after exposure to as little as 0.1 ml Rh positive blood. Others do not respond even after massive transplacental haemorrhage (TPH).[20,31] The transfer of IgG anti (D) antibodies from other to fetus takes place via the placenta. The anti (D) attaches to the erythrocytes of the fetus which are then destroyed in the reticulo endothelial system. This haemolytic process results in anaemia, erythroblastosis and the increased bilirubin production which is characteristic of haemolytic disease of the newborn.

PREVENTION OF IMMUNISATION

Several investigators have suggested that blocking the rhesus primary immunisation by injection of anti (D) antibodies could prevent the formation of antibodies.[4,8,10,20] Two groups, one in England and one in the United States, approached the problem in different ways but arrived at the same conclusions almost simultaneously.

The English group, from Liverpool, started with the observation that ABO incompatibility between mother and fetus offers protection against maternal Rh (D) immunisation.[3,8] The anti-A and anti-B isoagglutinins seem to be able to eliminate A or B cells and so prevent the production of antibodies

Experiments with Rh negative volunteers showed that chromium-51 labelled Rh positive cells were rapidly eliminated if anti (D) serum was given shortly after the injection of Rh positive blood.

The New York group based their work on the observations of Theobald Smith in 1909 that diphtheria immunisation by toxoid could be prevented if diphtheria antitoxin was given at the same time. In other words, passively administered antibody suppresses the active immune response.[10] Many clinical trials were performed by several groups of investigators. It appeared that with a standard dose of 200/300 µg anti (D) immunoglobulin, the post-delivery failure rate was 0.3-0.5% after the first Rh positive pregnancy with a further increase of 1 - 2% at the end of the next Rh positive pregnancy.[23,29] The expected immunisation rates in the absence of any therapy were 5% and 11% respectively.[28]

MECHANISM OF SUPPRESSION OF RH IMMUNISATION

Although the exact mechanism of action of anti (D) immunoprophylaxis is unknown, four possible attractive mechanisms of suppression of Rh immunisation should be considered:[1,2,7,31]

1. Rh antibody prevents the Rh (D) antigen from reaching the germinal centres of lymph nodes and spleen where potential immunocytes are produced.
2. Rh antibody may block or bind Rh antigenic determinants on red cell membranes so that no contact of the antigen with the surface receptors of the potential immunocytes occurs
3. Rh antibody may have a direct suppressive effect on the potential immunocytes.
4. Rh antibody shortens the arrival of D positive cells, causing their destruction in the spleen before they can reach the potential immunological responsive sites.

The amount of anti (D) immunoglobulin necessary to prevent active immunisation will depend on the volume of Rh positive cells circulating in the Rh negative subject. This suggests that anti (D) immunoglobulin prophylaxis does not act by modifying immune responses, but rather by a direct interaction with the D antigens on the red cell surface. An effective dose of anti D appears to shorten survival of (D) positive cells and anti (D) immunoglobulin seems to be effective even after the Rh positive cells erythrocytes have left the circulation.

This suggests that although the third and fourth mechanisms are probably the most important in preventing immunisation, they are not the only means, and an additional central working mechanism may play a role.

INDICATIONS FOR ANTI (D) IMMUNOPROPHYLAXIS

Post-Partum

In the majority of cases not more than 0.1 ml of fetal blood is found in the maternal circulation after parturition.[31] In approximately five percent of cases a transplacental haemorrhage of 5 ml or more is observed after delivery. Fetomaternal transfusion of more than 30 ml has been reported in 0.2 - 0.6% of births[1.28.31].

Pollock et al showed that doses of anti (D) immunoglobulin of 10 µgs and higher offer complete protection in cases of transplacental haemorrhage of 1 ml or less.[19] It is obvious that the routine administration of different doses of anti (D) immunoglobulin, based on the volume of TPH determined by the Kleihauer test would be highly impractical. Therefore, in most countries a standard dose of 200 - 300 µgs anti (D) immunoglobulin is administered to every non-immunised Rh (D) negative woman who delivers an Rh (D) positive child.

In Holland, the Rh prevention programme started in 1969. At first, due to a shortage of anti-D immunoglobulin only non-immunised Rh (D) negative women who were delivered of ABO compatible infants could be treated. In 1970 this immunoprophylaxis programme was expanded to include all non-immunised Rh (D) negative women giving birth to an Rh (D) positive baby, and a dose of 200 µg anti (D) immunoglobulin became standard.

Post-abortion

The general influence of abortion in the overall picture of Rh (D) immunisation has been difficult to evaluate. The incidence of TPH in spontaneous abortion has been estimated at about 6%.[16] In therapeutic abortion the incidence seems to be much higher; according to some authors up to 25%.[16,25] The frequency of TPH increases with the duration of the pregnancy. Pregnancy terminations from 12 weeks onwards are reported to give a TPH incidence of 16 - 40%.[25] Usually fetomaternal transfusion of not more than 0.1-0.2 ml is encountered,[11] a TPH exceeding 1 ml being a rare occurrence.

In retrospective studies, 3 - 4% Rh (D) negative women are immunised by a first pregnancy ending in early abortion.[9,11] Little is known about the incidence of immunisation in second trimester abortion but Freda et al estimate that the risk of immunisation increases proportionally with gestational age to approximately 9% at three months and beyond.[9] Nowadays it is common practice to provide women undergoing therapeutic abortion with anti (D) immunoglobulin. In early abortion a dose of 50–75 μgs seems sufficient. In second trimester abortion a dose of 200–300 μgs is to be recommended. Anti (D) immunoprophylaxis following spontaneous abortion is still too frequently neglected, and the Rh prevention programme in many countries fails in this respect.[5,30]

DURING PREGNANCY

Ante partum immunisation

The presence of small amounts of fetal red cells in the maternal circulation during pregnancy indicates the risk of subsequent antibody formation. Some investigators estimate the risk of immunisation at 0.5–1.5%.[7] In other studies a much higher percentage is found.[31] The use of very sensitive autoanalyser antibody detection techniques in some studies may be responsible for these higher frequencies.

As ninety percent of antepartum transplacental haemorrhages occur after 28 weeks of pregnancy, administration of 200–300 μgs anti (D) immunoglobulin in the 28th and 34th weeks of gestation has been advocated.[1,2,13,31] This would mean that at least three times the present amount of anti (D) immunoglobulin would be required for each pregnancy, involving a tremendous increase in the cost of Rh prevention, most of it unnecessarily. In most European countries parents tend to limit their families to two or three children. As immunisation occurring during the first pregnancy is generally benign, immunoprophylaxis during pregnancy will have only a limited value in terms of lowering perinatal mortality due to HDN. It was for this reason that Rh prevention committees in the U.K. and in the Netherlands, among others, decided against administration of anti (D) immunoglobulin in the antenatal period.

Amniocentesis

Fetomaternal haemorrhage after amniocentesis has been reported by several investigators. Usually the incidence of fetomaternal haemorrhage in second trimester amniocentesis is less than 15%. In third trimester amniocenteses the incidence is reported to be much higher, sometimes as high as 30%.[12,14] The incidence is lower when there is a posterior placenta and highest in the case of an anterior placenta. Accordingly, all Rh (D) negative women should receive immunoprophylaxis following amniocentesis either early or late in pregnancy.

External version

The administration of anti (D) immunoglobulin following external version of breech to cephalic presentation is a controversial issue. Since some authors have reported small transplacental haemorrhages it may be wise to perform a Kleihauer test before and after the procedure.[12,15,26] In the event of transplacental haemorrhage anti (D) immunoglobulin should be administered.

Abdominal trauma during pregnancy

Fetomaternal transfusions have been demonstrated in cases of abdominal trauma during pregnancy. A Kleihauer test is therefore recommended.

Blood loss in the third trimester of pregnancy

Placenta praevia, abruption or bleeding from the margin of the placenta may cause transplacental haemorrhage.[22] If fetal red blood cells are detected by the Kleihauer test, anti (D) immunoglobulin should be administered.

Fetal or intra partum death and the birth of an anaemic child

When a fetal or intra partum death occurs it is useful to count the fetal erythrocytes in the maternal circulation because fetal mortality is sometimes caused by massive transplacental haemorrhage.[22] This also applies to anaemia in the newborn child.

Failure of immunoprophylaxis

Failures can be divided into two categories: utilization failure and failure to prevent immunization.

Utilization failure

This is the failure to make adequate use of immunoprophylaxis. In the U.S. and the U.K. about 20% of the women at risk were still not being treated in 1978.[5,30] In Holland the use of anti (D) immunoglobulin after parturition and induced abortion is 98 - 100%,*but immunoprophylaxis after spontaneous abortion has not yet entered common practice.

The main reasons why not all women at risk of Rh (D) immunization get immunoprophylaxis are:

1. Poor organisation.
2. Negligence on the part of doctors and midwives.
3. Faulty Rh bloodtyping in mother and/or child.
4. The fact that anti (D) immunoglobulin is not administered after spontaneous or induced abortions in the at risk population.

*Data from the Central Laboratory of the Dutch Red Cross, Amsterdam

Failure to prevent immunisation

Failure to prevent immunisation following administration of Rh (D) immunoglobulin within 72 hours post partum in non-sensitised Rh women who give birth to a Rh positive infant occurs in 0.5–1.5% (0.5% new immunisations per annum in the Netherlands*).[5,7,31] The reasons for this are:

1. Antepartum immunisation.
2. Maternal-fetal transplacental haemorrhage (grandmother theory)
3. Massive transplacental haemorrhage during or after delivery.

To explain the development of the immunisation during a first Rh (D) positive pregnancy, immunisation due to the passage of Rh positive maternal cells to an Rh negative infant at the time of birth has been proposed and administration of Rh anti (D) immunoglobulin to Rh negative babies born to Rh (D) positive mothers has even been advised.[6] Although there is some reason to believe that this mechanism may be operative on occasion, the evidence is equivocal.[17,21,24]

Massive transplacental haemorrhage

Pollock showed that 10 µg Rh anti (D) immunoglobulin results in complete protection against transplacental haemorrhages of up to 1 ml.[19] Therefore, the standard dose of 200 µg anti (D) immunoglobulin would be adequate to prevent immunisation in transplacental haemorrhages of 20 ml or less. Transplacental haemorrhages of 20 ml or more are reported by some authors to occur in 0.2% and by others in 0.6% of deliveries.[1,31]

Zipursky has pointed out that a massive transplacental haemorrhage usually seen in association with manual removal of the placenta or with caesarian section, may often occur during the delivery of a normal non-anaemic child. He and others suggest that a Kleihauer test should be done as a routine procedure after every delivery at risk.[23,31]

Conclusions

Although the incidence of Rh immunisation has been considerably reduced, the lowest possible level has yet to be attained. To reach this goal, all Rh (D) negative women must receive anti (D) immunoglobulin after abortion or delivery of an Rh positive child. A dose of 200 µg of anti (D) immunoglobulin would seem to be adequate.

Attention should be focussed primarily on utilisation failures rather than on

*Data from the Central Laboratory of the Dutch Red Cross, Amsterdam

the failures of anti (D) immunoglobulin. Immunoprophylaxis antepartum has a very low cost to benefit ratio and does not appear to be beneficial, at least not in the Netherlands. Performing Kleihauer tests as a routine measure after every delivery at risk may have some influence on lowering the incidence of immunisation and should therefore be considered. Even when the lowest feasible level of Rh (D) immunisation is reached there will still be some cases of haemolytic disease.

It is of the utmost importance that obstetricians and paediatricians remain on the alert to the actual dangers of Rh immunisation, which have not disappeared, even though their frequency has been reduced. Centralisation of treatment for cases of immunisation has proved to be the most effective way to reduce perinatal mortality and morbidity in those patients where immunoprophylaxis has failed.

Summary

Ten years after the institution of the Rh (D) immunisation programme in Holland, the rate of new Rh immunisations appears to have been reduced from 3.5% to 0.5% per year. Failure of immunoprophylaxis is due mainly to immunisation during the first Rh positive pregnancy, massive transplacental haemorrhage and the fact that anti (D) immunoglobulin is not administered following spontaneous abortion. Measures to promote a further reduction of the immunisation frequency are discussed.

REFERENCES

1. Bowman, J.M.: Suppression of Rh isoimmunization. A review. Obstet. and Gynec. 52:385, 1978.
2. Bowman, J.M., Chown, B., Lewis, M., Pollock, J. and H. Kaita: Rh immunization in Manitoba 1963-1974. Ann.roy.coll.Phys.Surg.Canad. 9:47, 1976.
3. Clarke, C.A.: Bloodgroup incompatibility between mother and fetus. Clin.Sci. 43:1, 1972.
4. Clarke, C.A., Donohoe, W.T.A., McConnell, R.B., Woodrow, J.C., Finn, R., Krevans, J.R., Kulke, W., Lehane, D. and P.M. Sheppard: Further experimental studies on the prevention of Rh haemolytic disease. Brit.med.J. i:979, 1963.
5. Clarke, C. and A.G.W. Whitfield: Death from Rh haemolytic disease in England and Wales in 1977: accuracy of records and assessment of anti-D prophylaxis. Brit.med.J. 1:1665, 1979.
6. Cohen, F. and W.W. Zuelzer: The transplacental passage of maternal erythrocytes into the fetus. Am.J.Obstet.Gynec. 93:566, 1965.
7. Eklund, J: Prevention of Rh immunization in Finland. A national study 1969-1977. Acta paediat.scand. suppl.:274, 1978.
8. Finn, R., Clarke, C.A., Donohoe, W.T.A., McConnell, R.B., Sheppard, P.M., Lehane, D. and W. Kulke: Experimental studies on the prevention of Rh haemolytic disease. Brit.med.J. 1:1486, 1961.
9. Freda, V.J., Gorman, J.G., Galen, R.S. and N. Treacy: The threat of Rh immunisation from abortion. Lancet 147, 1970.
10. Freda, V.J., Gorman, J.G. and W. Pollock: Successful prevention of experimental Rh sensitization in man with anti-Rh $gamma_2$globulin antibody preparation. Transfusion 4:26, 1964.
11. Goldman, J.A. and B. Eckerling: Prevention of Rh immunization after abortion with anti-Rh(D) immunoglobulin. Obstet.and.Gynec. 40:366, 1972.
12. Goldstein, A.I. and F. Pezzlo: Fetal-maternal hemorrhage after amniocentesis: incidence, degree and ramifications. Int.J.Gynec. and Obstet. 16:187, 1978.
13. Harrison, K.L.: Fetal cell counting as an evaluation of Rh prophylaxis with antenatally administered anti-Rh(D) gamma-globulin. Transfusion 17:647, 1977.
14. Hill, L.M., Platt, L.D. and B. Kellog: Rh sensitization after genetic amniocentesis. Obstet. and Gynec. 56:459, 1980.
15. Kleihauer, E., Braun, H. and K. Betke: Demonstation von fetalem Hämoglobin in den Erythrocyten eines Blutausstrichs. Klin.Wschr. 35:637, 1957.

16. Matthews, C.D. and A.E.B. Matthews: Transplacental haemorrhage in spontaneous and induced abortion. Lancet 1:694, 1969.

17. Perrault, R.: Low concentration red cell antibodies, Rh D. Thesis, Uppsala University, 1972.

18. Pollock, A.: Transplacental haemorrhage after external cephalic version. Lancet I:612, 1972.

19. Pollock, W., Ascari, W.Q., Kochesky, R.J., O'Connor, R.R., Ho, T.Y. and D. Tripodi: Studies on Rh prophylaxis: relationship between doses of anti Rh and size of antigenic stimulus. Transfusion 11:333, 1971.

20. Queenan, J.T. and J. Schneider: Practical clinical aspects of Rh-prophylaxis. J.perinat.Med. 1:223, 1973.

21. Ramos de Almeida, J.M. and L. Rosado: Rh blood group of grandmother and incidence of erythroblastosis. Arch.Dis.Childh. 47:609, 1972.

22. Renaer, M., Putte, I.vd. and C. Vermeijlen: Massive fetomaternal haemorrhage as a cause of perinatal mortality and morbidity. Europ.J.Obstet.and Gynec. 6/3:125, 1976.

23. Report to the Medical Research Council by the working party on the use of anti-D immunoglobulin for the prevention of isoimmunisation of Rh-negative women during pregnancy; controlled trial of various anti-D dosages in suppression of Rh sensitisation following pregnancy. Brit.med.J. 1:75, 1974.

24. Taylor, J.F.: Sensitization of Rh negative daughters by their Rh positive mothers. New.Engl.J.Med. 276:547, 1967.

25. Voigt, J.C. and R.P. Britt: Feto-maternal haemorrhage in therapeutic abortion. Brit.med.J. 4:395, 1969.

26. Vos, G.H.: The effect of external version on antenatal immunization by the Rh factor. Vox Sang. 12:390, 1967.

27. Woodrow, J.C., Clarke, C.A., Donohoe, W.T.A., Finn, R., McConnell, R.B., Sheppard, P.M., Lehane, D., Roberts, F.M. and T.M.D. Gimlette: Mechanism of Rh prophylaxis: An experimental study on specificity of immunosuppression. Brit.med.J. 2:57, 1975.

28. Woodrow, J.C. and W.T.A. Donohoe: Rh-immunisation by pregnancy; results of a survey and their relevance to prophylactic therapy. Brit.med.J. 4:139, 1968.

29. World Health Organisation: Prevention of Rh Sensitisation. Wld Hlth Org.techn.Rep.Ser. 468:1, 1971.

30. Wysowski, D.K., Flint, J.W., Goldberg, M.F. and F.A. Conell: Rh hemolytic disease: Epidemiologic Surveillance in the United States, 1968 to 1975. J.Amer.med.Ass. 242:1376, 1979.

31. Zipurski, A.: Rh hemolytic disease of the newborn; the disease eradicated by immunology. Clin.Obstet.and Gynec. 20:759, 1977.

----

3. DISCUSSION

moderator: G. GARRATTY

A.S. KHALIFA (Cairo, Egypt): In August 1980, there was a symposium at the International Haematology Meeting in Montreal in which failure of anti (D) prophylaxis was discussed. The conclusion reached was that there was a 1.6% failure rate. The cost of giving anti (D) after the 28th week of gestation was given as (U.S.) $100,000 per baby saved. This point was made by both British and Canadian workers attending that meeting. They give anti (D) to any Rh negative mother irrespective. It is given at the 28th week of gestation and immediately following delivery at a cost of $100,000 per life saved.
T.J. WALSH (Dublin, Ireland): With reference to the production of anti (D) and the amount of anti (D) required from the number of donors: in Ireland we use the intravenous method to prepare anti (D). We are able to prepare some 8,000 doses from 12 immunised male donors who each give something like eight plasmaphereses per year or 40 litres of plasma. Production of anti (D) by this method has advantages: we can get away with using 100 µgs, recovery from the starting pool is probably much better, and fewer donors are put at risk in terms of immunisation - which is an important consideration. We have seen two donors making anti-S, even in our small pool.
G. GARRATTY: Are the clinical side effects just as low with the intravenous preparations? What sort of side effects were seen?
T J WALSH: We have seen only two instances of side effects, two reaction in ten years since the introduction of this programme. They were mild allergic reactions, very mild, and both easily dealt with. The results in terms of prophylaxis were very satisfactory too. We find a failure rate of less than 0.5%.
G. GARRATTY: The 72 hours following delivery for giving the anti (D) - in America at any rate - seems a very arbitrary figure. Has Professor Bennebroek Gravenhorst any experience or can he relate the experience of other workers on how late the anti (D) can be given?

J. BENNEBROEK GRAVENHORST: To achieve a very high success rate it should be given before the 72 hours, but some investigators have noted partial success even when a dose of the anti (D) immunoglobulin has been given after two or three weeks. That is why when immunoglobulin has to be given for amniocentesis in Rh negative women, if the amniocentesis has to be repeated after a week or two we advise that it is not necessary to give an additional dose of anti (D) immunoglobulin. The circulating time of the immunoglobulin is such that there will be enough immunoglobulin left to prevent small fetomaternal transfusions. But as the period lengthens, the concentrations of immunoglobulin will decrease and only small fetomaternal transfusions will be neutralised.

G. GARRATTY: Has Prof. Bennebroek Gravenhorst or any of the other participants any experience of treating ladies who have enzyme-only or AutoAnalyzer-only reacting antibodies at delivery?

J. BENNEBROEK GRAVENHORST: No. In Holland we have no experience of that, but it has been reported in the literature. Up to now the results have been rather controversial.

G. GARRATTY: I know that Dr Bowman has reported treating 30 such patients and believes that the immunisation cannot be stopped; that once they have started producing even an enzyme-only antibody it cannot be stopped. But I believe that it is controversial and I wondered if anybody had had any direct experience.

J. BENNEBROEK GRAVENHORST: That is right, and he claims that in the next pregnancy the haemolytic disease will be less severe. But it is a controversial issue still.

G. GARRATTY: Are enzyme autoanalyzers used in the Netherlands for the detection of antibodies? If so, what is the general practice? Do the physicians usually give the Rh IgG or not?

M.A.M. OVERBEEKE (Amsterdam, Netherlands): We do not use an autoanalyser but we do use enzyme tests. But it is the same thing. If we find antibodies only in the enzyme tests we can stop them. When we find antibodies only in the enzyme tests we still give anti (D) postnatally because it is better to give it and to stop them.

J BENNEBROEK GRAVENHORST: But we do not have much experience as yet.

R.L. McSHINE (Groningen, Netherlands): We have just started to use an autoanalyzer for the detection of antibodies. Our experience is very limited but it has been developed.

J. BENNEBROEK GRAVENHORST: The problem is that the autoanalyzer is a very sensitive method and it has not yet been proven that the antibodies that are found by using it are really harmful.

M.M. KERR (Glasgow, U.K.): May I ask for an explanation for the high failure rate with spontaneous abortions?

J. BENNEBROEK GRAVENHORST: The utilisation rate? It has not yet been done in Holland. Up to now there has not been a programme for it. We have just started to make ampoules with a lower dose, 75 μgs. We hope to start a campaign very shortly to have anti (D) immunoglobulin administered after spontaneous abortions, but there are a lot of problems. At what time should the anti (D) immunoglobulin be given? Should it be administered at the point where the woman starts to lose blood? Should it be given before or after curettage? What about the women who lose blood for two, three or four weeks and then finally abort? Then there is a sizable group of women who lose blood for two or three weeks but the outcome is not abortion and their pregnancies go on in the normal way. Those are rather difficult problems.

We would advise giving anti (D) immunoglobulin to every Rh negative woman who has a spontaneous abortion because that group can be identified.

M.M. KERR: Would the woman who has a spontaneous abortion in Holland always come into hospital?

J. BENNEBROEK GRAVENHORST: No. That is another point. We have to get through to the general physicians.

J.G. JOLLY (Chandigahr, India): In her interesting presentation, Dr. Reerink-Brongers stated that Rh immunisation in first pregnancy is recorded in a couple of cases. This is well established, but was it investigated and what could have been the result in that particular series?

J. BENNEBROEK GRAVENHORST: If I may answer that question. There are two possible reasons. Firstly, there may have been small fetomaternal transfusions, small fetomaternal bleeds during pregnancy, perhaps starting at 16 weeks, although in about ninety percent they will only start after 28 weeks of pregnancy. Then there is already some immunisation at the start of delivery, and the transplacental haemorrhage during delivery serves as a means of immunisation. That is why sometimes during pregnancy antibodies are encountered, and sometimes after a very short period following delivery.

The second possibility is the "grandmother theory". An Rh negative woman has been sensitised by maternal-fetal transfusion during her own fetal life, during the time that she herself spent in her own mother's uterus. A maternal-fetal transfusion occurred during her own delivery and this is the reason for immunisation in early childhood or during the first months of life. There are some indications that this might be true in a very small percentage of immunisations; not more than maybe 0.1% of those women at risk.

----

1. HAEMOLYTIC DISEASE OF THE NEWBORN: AN OVERVIEW OF THE PRINCIPLES OF THERAPY

J.O. FORFAR

INTRODUCTION

It is generally accepted that the term haemolytic disease of the newborn (HDN) covers two particular states of immunological incompatibility between mother and fetus, namely Rh and ABO blood group incompatibility.

A THERAPEUTIC PERSPECTIVE

Prevention is better than cure and one of the widely hailed advances in

Figure 1

HAEMOLYTIC DISEASE OF THE NEWBORN

NEONATAL DEATHS PER 1000 LIVE BIRTHS

England and Wales

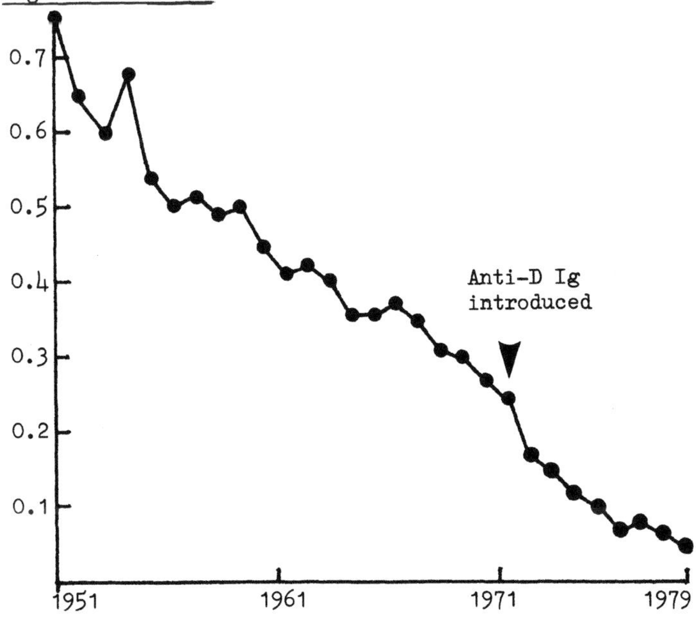

preventive medicine in recent years has been the prevention of the possible damaging effects of Rh incompatibility by the administration at birth of anti-D Ig to Rh negative mothers who are delivered of an Rh positive infant. Anti-D Ig has not, however, been the sole factor in the improvement in the incidence of and outlook for HDN. Figures 1 and 2 show that there was a significant improvement in liveborn and stillbirth mortality rates attributable to

Figure 2

HAEMOLYTIC DISEASE OF THE NEWBORN

STILLBIRTHS PER 1000 TOTAL BIRTHS

England and Wales

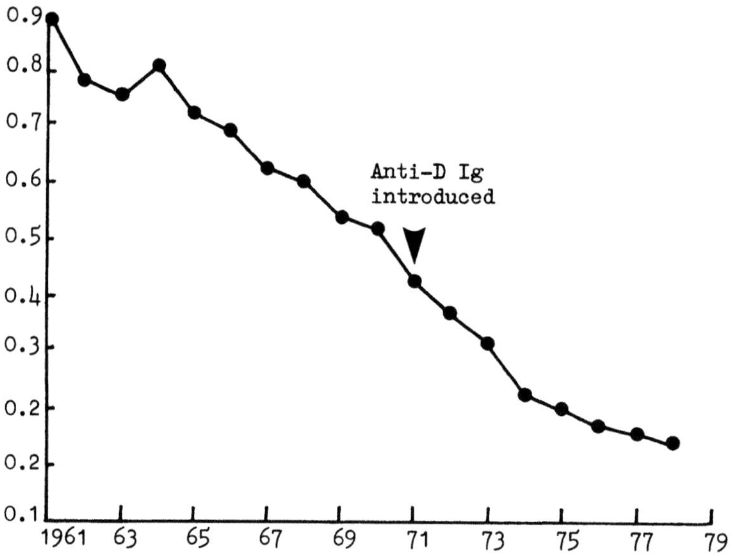

HDN before anti-D Ig was introduced. Figure 3 shows the combined mortality (stillbirths + neonatal deaths) experienced in respect of HDN for the ten years before the general introduction of anti-D Ig in 1971 and the subsequent mortality experienced. Thus, genetic counselling by clinicians and geneticists, better obstetric management of the pregnant mother and better paediatric management of the affected infant seem likely to have played at least as important a part in the improvement in HDN as anti-D Ig and still have an important role to play.

Effective as is prophylaxis with anti-D Ig given just after delivery it is not completely protective. One to three per cent (mean 1.7%) of women who have received anti-D Ig develop antibodies[1] related probably to factors such as

Figure 3

HAEMOLYTIC DISEASE OF THE NEWBORN

STILLBIRTHS + NEONATAL DEATHS PER 1000 TOTAL BIRTHS

England and Wales

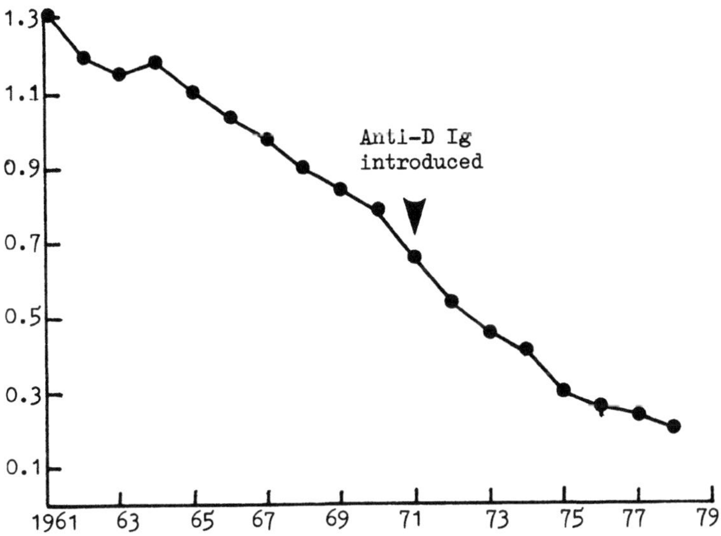

previously unrecognised abortions, obstetric procedures during pregnancy (such as amniocentesis or external version), abdominal injury during pregnancy or massive transplacental haemorrhage at birth which 'overwhelms' the amount of anti-D Ig given. In addition, at the present time, as many mothers develop anti-D antibodies because there has been failure to administer anti-D Ig.

The benefit conferred by anti-D Ig is not all or nothing. There is evidence that in Rh positive babies born to mothers who develop Rh antibodies despite having been given anti-D Ig HDN is likely to be less severe than in babies born to mothers who have not been given anti-D Ig.[8,13]

CURRENT SIZE OF THE PROBLEM

Rh Incompatibility

In Britain today for every thousand live-born infants delivered per annum there are three cases of HDN and there might be half that number if a fully effective programme of anti-D Ig administration was in operation (Table I). Twenty to thirty per cent of infants suffering from Rh incompatibility require exchange transfusion, ie, 1 in 1500 to 1 in 1000 liveborn infants (Table II) and

TABLE I

PREVALENCE OF HDN
DUE TO Rh INCOMPATIBILITY

	Per Million Population	Per Thousand Live Births
All susceptible treated with anti-D Ig*	20	1.5
1977/78 prevalence (U.K.)** (= x2)	40	3.0

*MRC trial (Brit.med.J., 1974)

**Based on: Clarke & Whitfield (1979)
Tovey (1980)

TABLE II

EXCHANGE TRANSFUSION IN RH AND ABO HDN

Rh	1/1000 live births
ABO	0.5/1000 live births
Rh and ABO	1.5/1000 live births

∴ @ 2 exchanges per exchanged infant
= 3/1000 live births

about two per cent of affected liveborn infants, say 1 in 50,000, die. Two to three times as many infants are stillborn due to Rh incompatibility as are liveborn and die from this cause (Table III),[3,4] ie, 1 in 12,500 fetuses are stillborn or die as newborn infants in the early neonatal period as a result of Rh incompatibility. These Rh deaths represent a very small proportion of perinatal deaths.

TABLE III

PERINATAL DEATHS FROM Rh HDN

(per total births)

Liveborn	1/50,000)	
	)	1/12,500
Stillborn	3/50,000)	
All perinatal deaths		200/12,500

ABO Incompatibility

The position quantitatively regarding ABO incompatibility is more difficult to define. In 20 per cent of pregnancies there is mother/child ABO incompatibility and the incidence of affected infants has been put at 1 - 3 per cent of all liveborn infants.[2,9,] Thus at 2 per cent, or 20 per 1000 live births the incidence of ABO HDN is seven times commoner among liveborn infants than HDN due to Rh incompatibility. The incidence, however, is somewhat arbitrary due to the different criteria adopted for diagnosis. Cases requiring exchange transfusion are a more definitive group related to the need for one of the major forms of therapy. The current position in Edinburgh is that for every two infants transfused on account of Rh disease one is transfused on account of ABO incompatibility (Table II).

From both causes, therefore, 2 - 3 infants in every 2000 delivered would be exchange-transfused. At an average of two exchanges per infant this means 2 - 3 exchanges per 1000 infants or 10 - 15 per year in a unit serving 5000 deliveries per annum, (or one per month on account of Rh and ABO incompatibility.

THE THERAPEUTIC TEAM

The effective management of HDN depends on the coordinated contributions of a number of people, on a mother educated to seek medical help early in her pregnancy; on a general practitioner alert to the need for early determination of the mother's and possibly the father's blood group; on an obstetrician who supervises the mother throughout her pregnancy, watching her antibody status (at say, 12, 24 and 34 weeks), effecting her delivery and assessing her need for the prophylactic administration of anti-D Ig; on a haematologist, a biochemist and a blood transfusion service to carry out the necessary investigations and if required provide the necessary blood for transfusion; and on a paediatrician who effectively evaluates, and if necessary treats, the affected infant.

EVALUATION OF THE PROBLEM

Clinical judgements enter in the management of HDN but the evaluation of the disease is peculiarly dependent on specific laboratory criteria.

During Pregnancy

We require to know the Rh and ABO grouping of the mother, whether she has antibodies and if so their titre. Her previous history and her Rh antibody titre in the present pregnancy may determine the further investigation by amniocentesis. Amniocentesis is likely to be indicated when there has been Rh disease in the previous pregnancy resulting in a stillbirth or a severely hydropic infant, or when in the previous pregnancy the antibody titre rises higher than 1 in 8. Amniocentesis has its major use from the 26th week of pregnancy until about the 35th. Based on the optical density (optical density difference) of the amniotic fluid so may the need for intrauterine transfusion or for early induction of labour be indicated. Decisions regarding intrauterine transfusion lie primarily in the province of the obstetrician. Decisions regarding induction of labour are joint obstetric/paediatric decisions. They involve a balance of judgement between the desirability of induction with a view to avoiding further intrauterine damage to the fetus and the undesirability of induction in terms of the increased risk of hyaline membrane disease. In striking a correct balance a consideration of the lecithin/spinglmyelin ratio as well as the optical density changes in the liquor will assist in decision making.

Fetomaternal ABO incompatibility is unlikely to be capable of diagnosis during pregnancy. Some years ago in Edinburgh we believed that examination of the mother's blood for anti-A and anti-B haemolysins gave a useful indication that the newborn infant would suffer from the effects of ABO incompatibility if haemolysins were found to be present. Recent re-evaluation of the results obtained over a number of years has shown that there is a very poor correlation between the presence of haemolysins in the mother's blood in pregnancy and clinical ABO incompatibility in the newborn infant. We have now abandoned this diagnostic procedure.

Postnatally

The routine evaluation on the cord blood of the infant at birth will include determination of the Rh and ABO grouping, a direct Coombs' test, a haemoglobin estimation and a serum bilirubin level. These are the tests which supply the criteria for management of both Rh and ABO incompatibility. Determination of the reticulocyte and the erythroblast counts, popular in the past, is now seldom employed.

With Rh incompatibility the timescale for action is likely to be short and therapeutic procedures may have to be instituted on the results of cord blood determinations alone or on the results of haemoglobin and serum bilirubin estimations on peripheral blood carried out at 6 or 12-hourly intervals. Table IV indicates the criteria of severity applicable in these early days; later when the hyperbilirubinaemia risk has passed haemoglobin estimation alone is the criterion determining action.

TABLE IV

HAEMOLYTIC DISEASE OF NEWBORN:
CRITERIA OF SEVERITY AND MANAGEMENT ACTION

Grade of Severity	Hb (g/dl)	Serum Bilirubin (μmol/l)	Likely Action
Severe	< 10	> 70	Exchange transfusion
Moderate	10 - 13	51 - 70	Monitor HB and serum bilirubin 6-hourly*
Mild	> 13	> 30 - 50	Monitor Hb and serum bilirubin 12-hourly*

*Exchange transfusion if within first week of life
Hb falls below 8 g/dl; or if at any time
serum bilirubin exceeds 300 μmol/l, or on plotting graphically
appears likely to do so.

The diagnosis of ABO incompatibility depends on the recognition that the mother is Group O and the baby is Group A or B and exhibiting a degree of jaundice exceeding 230 µmol/l. The Coombs' test may be positive but more often than not is negative. There is no specific confirmatory test for ABO incompatibility.

CRITERIA FOR MANAGEMENT

Rh Incompatibility

Where a fetus is affected as a result of Rh incompatibility it is quite likely that on the basis of the mother's Rh grouping, her past history and the detection of antibodies the diagnosis of the Rh incompatibility will have been made during pregnancy and will be confirmed at birth by the finding of a positive Coombs' test on cord blood. The major problem is likely to be the gauging of the severity of the disease and relating that to an appropriate form of therapy. Table IV gives an indication of the ranges (cord blood) of the two valid yardsticks of measurement in relation to severity, haemoglobin and serum bilirubin levels. Haemoglobin and serum bilirubin have to be considered separately. They are not related in any absolute way. Jaundice can occur in infants whose haemoglobin levels are within the normal range because of the variation between infants in the efficiency of hepatic bilirubin conjugation and excretion. Table IV also indicates the likely action necessary for the varying degrees of severity. After the first week of life a top-up transfusion is likely to be adequate in terms of a low haemoglobin level (< 10 g/dl).

Critical levels of serum bilirubin (indirect acting) are not of course solely dependent on absolute figures. With the low birthweight infant in whom the blood brain barrier is less efficient and brain cells probably more susceptible to damage, criteria for exchange transfusion would be set at a somewhat lower level of serum bilirubin. States of acidosis may also alter the efficiency of the blood brain barrier so that serum bilirubin levels that might otherwise be considered safe are no longer so. Diminished bilirubin binding due to hypoalbuminaemia or competition for binding sites by drugs such as salicylates also means that at lower serum bilirubin levels the infant is at risk of kernicterus and exchange transfusion is likely to be indicated.

ABO incompatibility

ABO incompatibility creates only two significant clinical problems requiring therapy, namely hyperbilirubinaemia and anaemia. Hyperbilirubinaemia usually reaches its maximum on the 3rd or 4th day of life. With the use of phototherapy only about 1 in 20 - 40 affected infants, (ie, about 1 in 1000 to 1 in 2000 of all newborn infants - Table II) experiences a level of 340μmol/l at which exchange transfusion would be considered necessary.

Anaemia associated with ABO incompatibility usually appears between two and six weeks after birth and is seldom severe.

Other Blood Group Incompatibilities

As a result of blood transfusion, and less commonly as a result of feto-maternal haemorrhage, maternal antibodies to the so-called 'minor' blood groups such as c, e, E, Duffy, Kell, Kidd, M or S may develop. As the mother will also often be Rh positive these antibodies may not come to light during pregnancy and may be revealed postnatally by the clinical state of the infant accompanied by a positive Coombs' test. Clinical management is along the same lines as that for the other types of HDN.

THERAPY

Exchange Transfusion

In Rh incompatibility exchange transfusion using Group O Rh negative blood fulfils the three functions of removing susceptible Rh positive red cells and replacing them with non-susceptible Rh negative red cells, removing bilirubin, and removing antibody. An exchange of 200 ml/kg will replace approximately 90 percent of the recipient's blood, 100 ml/kg 70 percent and 50 ml/kg 45 percent (Table V).[7] Where the removal of bilirubin is the primary object in exchange transfusion both volume and rate are important. Optimal figures are 200 ml/kg for volume and 1.8 ml/kg/minute for rate - which together give a transfusion time of approximately 2 hours (Table V).[5]

In an Rh affected infant who has received an exchange transfusion further anaemia and hyperbilirubinaemia may occur. A further fall in haemoglobin below the level of 8 g/dl or a further rise in serum bilirubin above 300 μmol/l or a rapid rise which indicates graphically the likelihood of reaching 300 μmol/l would be indications for another exchange transfusion. In severe cases of Rh HDN two, three or more exchanges may be required. If an infant suffering from ABO incompatibility requires exchange transfusion Group O blood of the same Rh group is usually used.

Exchange transfusion does of course have its risks. These include hypothermia, perforation of the umbilical vein, air embolism, septic thrombophlebitis with portal vein thrombosis, cytomegalovirus infection, hyperkalaemia, hypovolaemia and hypervolaemia; and according to the type of blood used, hyperglycaemia, reactive hypoglycaemia, disturbance of acid-base status and hypocalcaemia (with citrated blood) and hypocoagulability and elevation of free fatty acids causing reduction of bilirubin binding (with heparinised blood). The risk of exchange transfusion, varying greatly according to the state of the infant being transfused, has been estimated as ranging from 0.7 to 7 percent in terms of mortality.

TABLE V

EXCHANGE TRANSFUSION

Volume	@ 90% exchange	200 ml/kg
	@ 70% exchange	100 ml/kg
	@ 45% exchange	50 ml/kg
Rate:	1.8 ml/kg/minute	
Time:	200 ml/kg @ 1.8 ml/kg/min = 2 hours	

Late anaemia is a common occurrence both in infants who have been only mildly affected by HDN and have not required exchange transfusion and in more severely affected infants who have been treated by exchange transfusion. In such infants haemoglobin values usually fall steadily for the first 6 - 8 weeks of life and when the level falls below 10 g/dl top-up transfusion is usually indicated.

The striking fall over the past twenty years in the number of infants who have required exchange transfusion is illustrated in Figure 4.

Figure 4

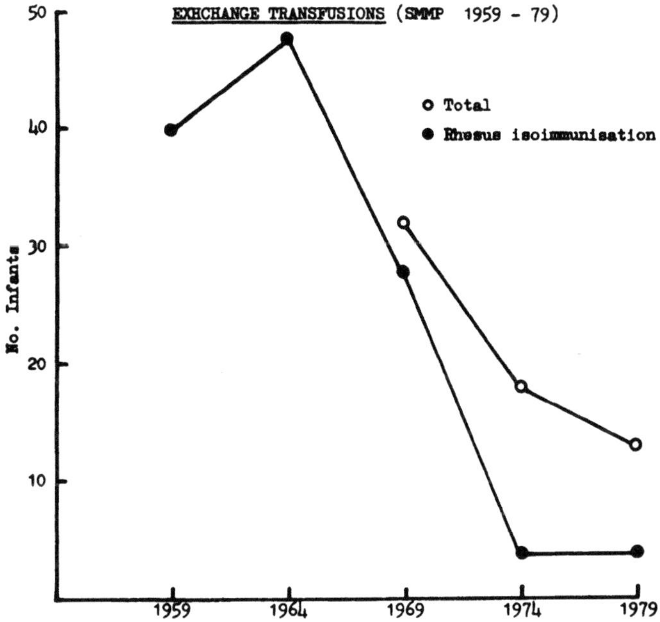

Phototherapy

Light of a certain wavelength (300-600 nm and particularly 425 - 475 nm) falling on the skin produces a photodecomposition of bile to an extent which lowers the serum bilirubin, or rather restrains its rise, to an amount of 15 - 35 µmol/l every 12 - 24 hours, or 1 µmol/l/hour. This degree of restraint clearly limits the effectiveness of phototherapy in Rh HDN where the concentration of bilirubin may be rising at a rate of 10 µmol/hour (Table VI). Phototherapy can, however, act as an adjunct to exchange transfusion, reducing the number necessary in infants affected by Rh incompatibility[10] or in a few cases enabling exchange transfusion to be avoided where serum bilirubin might otherwise have just exceeded the critical level.

Phototherapy has a more important role to play in the more slowly developing jaundice associated with ABO incompatibility. It reduces significantly the need for exchange transfusion in ABO incompatibility[6,11] but does not wholly remove the need for exchange transfusion.

In using phototherapy it is important to ensure that the light source emits light of the appropriate wavelength. Standard striplite tubes are of little value. Phototherapy also has its risks, particularly overheating and dehydration of the infant.

Phenobarbitone Therapy

Phenobarbitone, through hepatic mechanisms not fully understood, reduces hyperbilirubinaemia. It is most effective when given to the mother before birth. The drug can be administered to the mother for two weeks before delivery and to the infant for 3 - 4 days after birth, being given to the latter in a dosage of 5 mg/kg/day.

The exact role of phenobarbitone therapy in the treatment of HDN has not been established. It does not appear to be widely used but may have a place in reducing the number of exchange transfusions or in avoiding exchange transfusions where the criteria for these are only marginally met.

TABLE VI

PHOTOTHERAPY IN HDN

Reducing effect on rising serum bilirubin	= 1 μmol/l/hour
Possible rate of rise of serum bilirubin in Rh HDN	= 10 μmol/l/hour

----

REFERENCES

1. Medical Research Council: Report on the use of Anti-D Immunoglobulin for the Prevention of Isoimmunisation of Rh Negative Women during Pregnancy. Brit.med.J. 2:75, 1974.
2. Clarke, C.A.: Practical Effects of Blood Group Incompatibilities between Mother and Fetus. Brit.med.J. 2:90, 1972.
3. Clarke, C.A. and A.G.W. Whitfield: Deaths from Rhesus Haemolytic Disease in England and Wales in 1977: Accuracy of Records and Assessment of Anti-D Prophylaxis. Brit.med.J. 1:1665, 1979.
4. Clarke, C.A. and A.G.W. Whitfield: Deaths from Rhesus Haemolytic Disease in England and Wales in 1978: Accuracy of Records and Assessment of Anti-D Prophylaxis. Brit.med.J. 281:781, 1980.
5. Forfar, J.O., Keay, A.J., Elliott, W.D. and R.A. Cumming: Exchange Transfusion in Neonatal Hyperbilirubinaemia. Lancet 2:1131, 1958.
6. Kaplan, E., Herz, F., Sheye, E. and D. Robinson: Phototherapy in ABO Haemolytic Disease of the Newborn Infant. J.Pediat. 79:911, 1971.
7. Landow, E.M.: Volume Estimation for Partial Exchange Transfusion. J. Pediat. 95:490, 1979.
8. Mitchell, R., O'Donnell, R., Blair, R.G. and Blue: Antenatal Anti-D Prophylaxis. Lancet 2:798, 1980.
9. Mollison, P.L.: Blood Transfusion in Clinical Medicine, London, Blackwell, 1979.
10. Möller, J., and F. Ebbesen: Phototherapy in Newborn Infants with Severe Rhesus Haemolytic Disease. J.Pediat. 86:135, 1975.
11. Sisson, T.R.C., Kendall, N., Glauser, S.C., Knutson, S. and E. Bunyaviroch: Phototherapy of Jaundice in Newborn Infants. I. ABO Group Incompatibility. J.Pediat. 79:904, 1971.
12. Tovey, G.H.: Should Anti-D Immunoglobulin be given Antenatally? Lancet 2:466, 1980.
13. Tovey, L.A.D. and A.E. Robinson: Reduced Severity of Rh Haemolytic Disease after Anti-D Immunoglobulin Administration. Brit.med.J.4:320, 1975.

2. THE USE OF COMPONENT THERAPY IN THE NEWBORN

T.L. TURNER

Acquired coagulation defects in the newborn are uncommon and require a high degree of technical skill on the part of laboratory and clinical staff in their management. They occur more commonly in preterm infants in association with asphyxia, pulmonary hyaline membrane disease, low birthweight (LBW) and sepsis. In mature infants asphyxia and sepsis are the commonest provoking agents. Congenital coagulation defects are rare in the newborn infant and will not be discussed here. In the LBW infant a frequent terminal event is cerebral intraventricular haemorrhage (IVH) and it was whilst investigating this problem that a component policy evolved.

As in all investigations using coagulation studies it was necessary to

TABLE I

SUGGESTED 'NORMAL' VALUES

	Preterm	Term
Prothrombin time (PT), seconds	13 28	13 24
Thrombotest per cent	30 - 50	40 - 60
Partial thromboplastin time (PTT), seconds	35 - 100	40 - 60
Thrombin time, seconds	12 - 24	12 - 18
Reptilase time, seconds	18 - 36	18 - 30
Fibrinogen, g/l	1.0 - 3.5	1.5 - 3.5
Platelet count, x 10^9/l	100 - 400	150 - 400

These 'normal' values are given only as a guide. These values will also vary if capillary techniques are used.

establish a range of normal values and this was elaborated during a pilot study (Table 1). Coagulation screens were performed on a maximum 3 ml specimen of blood drawn from an indwelling umbilical or venous catheter taking care to avoid heparin contamination. Aliquots were contained in plastic tubes containing citrate (2 ml), EDTA (0.5 ml) and Trasylol (0.5 ml) and used to determine the prothrombin time (PT), Kaolin partial thromboplastin time (PTT), Thrombin time with and without the addition of protamine sulphate, and packed cell volume as described by Hardisty and Ingram.[2] Plasma fibrinogen concentration was assayed according to Ellis and Stransky.[1] The ethanol gelation test (EGT) was performed as described by Keiruff and Godall[3] and platelet count determined using a thrombocounter (Coulter Electronics Ltd). Commercial reagents were used to assay fibrin degradation products (FDP) (Thrombo-Wellcotest, Wellcome Reagents Ltd) and Reptilase time (Pentapharm Ltd) using methods described by the manufacturers.

In order to evaluate the efficacy of component therapy in sick newborn infants, and in particular those which were preterm, we entered into our study infants with one or more of the following coagulation abnormalities:

1. PT greater than 28 seconds
2. PTT greater than 100 seconds
3. Plasma fibrinogen concentration less than 1 g/l
4. Platelet count less than 100 x 10^9/l.

Infants who weighed less than 1500 gms and had a gestation of less than 34 weeks were entered into the trial and had their haemostatic screening performed as soon as possible after birth. If normal, the screen was repeated at 6 - 8 hour intervals. If abnormal haemostasis was detected at any time during the next 48 hours the infant was included in the trial of component therapy and was randomly allocated to control or treatment group using a closed envelope system.

Treatment was provided as indicated by the coagulation status using prothrombin complex concentrate as a source of Factors II, VII, IX and X containing approximately 25 times the normal plasma concentration of these factors and 10 µ/ml of heparin as a lyophilised powder in vials for reconstitution to 2 ml by the Scottish National Blood Transfusion Service Protein Fractionation Centre. Fibrinogen and Factor VIII were provided from single donor units of cryoprecipitate containing approximately 200 mg of fibrinogen and 80 units of Factor VIII. Platelet concentrate was also supplied as a single donor unit containing about 0.7 x 10^{11} platelets. All three blood products were screened for the presence of HB_sAg prior to use. Infants treated received the above blood products when appropriate using the same criteria as for entry into the trial. Prothrombin complex was given to infants with prolonged PT at a dose of 1 ml/kg. Low plasma fibrinogen or platelet count was treated with cryoprecipitate or platelet concentrate respectively, in each case a dose of 1 donor unit being given. A prolonged PTT was usually treated with cryoprecipitate but in some cases coagulation factor concentrate was deemed more appropriate. After treatment the screening procedure was repeated every 4 to 6 hours until a sustained correction was apparent. All infants were also given Vitamin K.

Results

Fifty-eight infants weighing less than 1500 g were investigated, 46 were found to have abnormal coagulation screens according to the criteria previously described. There were no significant differences in mean birthweight, gestation or age of entry between the infants allocated to treatment or control groups, nor was there any significant difference in mortality between the two groups; 13 (57%) and 16 (70%) of the treatment group died. Post mortem examination showed that whilst 8 of the 13 infants in the control group died of IVH only 5 of the treatment group did so, suggesting that treatment modified the course of the disease, although this did not reach statistical significance (X^2 = 1.6 p>0.2). Although there were five deaths in the 12 infants who maintained normal coagulation, none were due to IVH, validating our criteria for inclusion in the trial. Examination of the haemostatic abnormalities responsible for entry into the trial showed that in the treatment and control groups 7 infants had a single defect whilst 16 had a combination of defects. A higher incidence of combined defects was noted in infants who eventually died but did not reach statistical significance. A particularly fatal combination was that of abnormal PT and fibrinogen. The mean doses of the various blood products to correct these abnormalities was as shown on the accompanying table (Table II), and these treatments resulted in an appreciable correction of haemostasis as measured by laboratory tests. For example, the prothrombin time was returned to within the normal range in 23 of the 37 occasions it was used (Table III), whilst cryoprecipitate used for abnormal PTT returned the level to within normal range in 13 of 18 uses. Where cryoprecipitate was used for abnormal fibrinogen level concentrations this was effective in returning the plasma fibrinogen concentration to normal in 18 of 26 uses, whilst platelet concentrate returned the

TABLE II

MEAN DOSE FOR TREATMENT

Factor II, VII, IX and X Concentrate (ml)	1.54 ± 0.51
Cryoprecipitate for Abnormal PTT (ml)	12.8 ± 7.5
Cryoprecipitate for Abnormal Fibrinogen (ml)	12.9 ± 6.5
Platelet Concentrate (ml)	15.9 ± 4.9

Mean ± SD doses of therapeutic material

platelet count to within the normal range in 10 of 15 uses. Using the guidelines of returning coagulation parameters to those limits set for the trial, treatment was efficient in 80 percent of cases with a single defect and correction was achieved in 88 percent of those infants who survived. It was less effective (62%) in those infants who died.

TABLE III

EFFICIENCY OF TREATMENT

	Factors II, VII, IX & X Concentrate		Cryoprecipitate for Abnormal PTT		Cryoprecipitate for Abnormal Fibrinogen		Platelet Concentrate	
	Survivors		Survivors		Survivors		Survivors	
No. of Patients	4	14	3	11	6	12	-	5
Total Treatments	5	32	5	13	7	19	-	15
Efficient Treatments	5	18	3	10	7	11	-	10

Diagnosis of disseminated intravascular coagulation (DIC) is difficult in the newborn and we use a combination of decrease in platelet count or fibrinogen concentration accompanied by rising FDPs and red cell fragmentation as diagnostic features. We have attempted to treat identified infants with exchange transfusion using either ACD blood or heparinised blood and although responses were obtained, such measures alone are seldom sufficient to control the more severe forms of the disorder. We have also attempted management of DIC using heparinisation of the infant with an initial loading dose of 100 U/kg then 25 U/kg 6-hourly and augmented this with the use of component therapy without success. A very great deal of difficulty was experienced in maintaining appropriate control over the management of the infant despite the use of PTT and thrombin times as an index of efficacy.

In our experience cryoprecipitate and platelet concentrates are comparatively safe products particularly as in this case when prepared from single donations and given to recipients with a very low incidence of specific alloantibodies. As prothrombin complex concentrate is produced from large plasma pools there is an increased risk of hepatitis associated with its use. In our experience we have found no evidence of hepatitis on the follow-up study of surviving infants. The use of prothrombin complex concentrates has been associated with thrombo-embolic episodes particularly in certain higher risk groups, but in our experience, as there was no increase in the incidence of disseminated intravascular coagulation in the control and treatment groups in our study and no increased incidence of overt thrombosis this type of concentrate appears safe to use at doses of up to 30 U/kg. Our suggested scheme may be valuable as a guide to the management of preterm newborn infants with acquired coagulation defects (Table IV).

TABLE IV

FACTORS TESTED IN THE 'BASIC' COAGULATION INVESTIGATIONS AND THERAPEUTIC MATERIALS AVAILABLE[a]

Coagulation Test	Factors Tested	Therapeutic Material Containing Factors
Prothrombin Time (PT)	(I)[b],II,V,VII,IX,X	Prothrombin Complex (II,VII,IX,X) (factor concentrate)
Partial Thromboplastin Time(PTT)	I,II,V,VII,VIII, IX,X,XI,XII	Prothrombin Complex (II,VII,IX,X Cryoprecipitate (I,VIII)
Plasma Fibrinogen Concentration	I	Cryoprecipitate (I,VIII)
Platelet Count		Platelet Concentrate

a This table gives the therapeutic source of factors which will help correct deficiencies demonstrated by abnormal screening tests.

b Very low concentrations of Factor I will lengthen the Prothrombin Time.

Acknowledgement

None of this work would have been possible without the devoted efforts of the laboratory staff of the South-East Scotland Regional Blood Transfusion Service and the caring devotion of the Special Care Unit, Simpson Memorial Maternity Pavilion, nursing staff.

REFERENCES

1. Ellis, B.C. and A. Stransky: A quick and accurate method for the determination of fibrinogen in plasma. J.Lab.clin.Med. 58:447, 1961.

2. Hardisty, R.M. and G.I.G. Ingram: In Bleeding Disorders, Oxford, Blackwells Scientific Publications, 1965.

3. Keiruff, P. and H. Godall: Fibrinaemia in medical patients screened by the ethanol gelation test. Acta med. scand. 190:185, 1971.

----

3. METABOLIC EFFECTS OF EXCHANGE TRANSFUSION

N.R.C. ROBERTON

There can be no doubt that a standard double volume exchange transfusion, irrespective of the reason for which it is carried out imposes major physiological stresses on a newborn infant. If the blood used has been preserved by the addition of ACD or CPD the infant receives over the period of 90 - 120 minutes an infusion of 150 - 180 ml/Kg of a fluid with a high glucose content, low pH and bizarre electrolyte composition. This results in a rise in plasma levels of free fatty acid, insulin, glucogon, growth hormone, catecholamines, parathormone and TSH and a fall in levels of T3 and T4.

This review concentrates on the changes which take place in the plasma electrolytes, acid base status and oxygen carrying capacity of the infant during and after an exchange transfusion.

Electrolytes

The composition of the various donor bloods is given in Table I. Precise values are not known since there will always be some variation in composition due to the initial variability in the plasma chemistry of the blood donor. It can be seen however that non-heparinised blood has a very high sodium content and no ionised calcium. There is surprisingly little published data on potassium levels in the plasma of ACD and CPD blood of different ages but what there is does suggest that the potassium level rises on average by 0.5 - 1.0 mEq/l/day after the blood is drawn. However these are only average increases and potassium values in excess of 10 mEq/l may occur in some bloods sampled only 3 - 4 days after donation;[10] this fact is obviously germane to the sequelae of exchange transfusion using blood that is more than 24 - 48 hours old. The rate of rise of potassium in heparinised blood is undoubtedly faster than the rate of rise in ACD or CPD blood but precise values are not available.

What happens when fluids of this bizarre chemical composition are infused

TABLE I

COMPOSITION OF DIFFERENT TYPES OF DONOR BLOOD

	ACD Blood	CPD Blood	Heparinised Blood	
Na	160 - 177	165 - 170	140	mEq/l
K	4.0 + 1.0	5.4	4.0 (rapid rise)	mEq/l
HCO_3	> 6	14 - 18	23 27	mEq/l
pH	6.84 (fresh) 6.5 (2 days)	6.9 - 7.1	7.35 (?)	mEq/l
pCO_2	> 150	90 - 110	?	mm Hg
Ionized Ca	Nil	Nil	1.25	mEq/l
Glucose	350 - 450	350 - 450	70 - 120	mg%

into a neonate is also comparatively poorly documented. The paper by Tan and Tan[15] is the most recent data on what happens to plasma electrolytes in babies transfused with ACD blood 5 days old. Figures 1 and 2 show that despite the high sodium and potassium levels in the donor blood there was only a slight rise in both sodium and potassium levels in the infant's plasma, and that these fell to the pre-exchange levels within 4 - 6 hours of the procedure ending. This data is in line with the older literature showing comparatively little change in the plasma electrolytes despite the use of donor blood with very high sodium and potassium values.[1]

The lack of change in the infant's plasma sodium, potassium and chloride following exchange transfusion is perhaps not too surprising when one considers the relative proportion of the total body pool of a given electrolyte which is present in the plasma compared with other body fluid compartments or in the body tissues. However, it should be noted that most of the published work on plasma electrolyte changes in infants following exchange transfusion is of studies on full term babies and there is little or no comparable data on the effect on sick infants, particularly those of short gestation, in whom the ability to regulate electrolyte milieu is seriously impaired. Yet, clinical experience suggests that it is in just such infants that potentially fatal metabolic

Figure 1

PLASMA SODIUM LEVELS BEFORE, DURING AND AFTER EXCHANGE TRANSFUSION

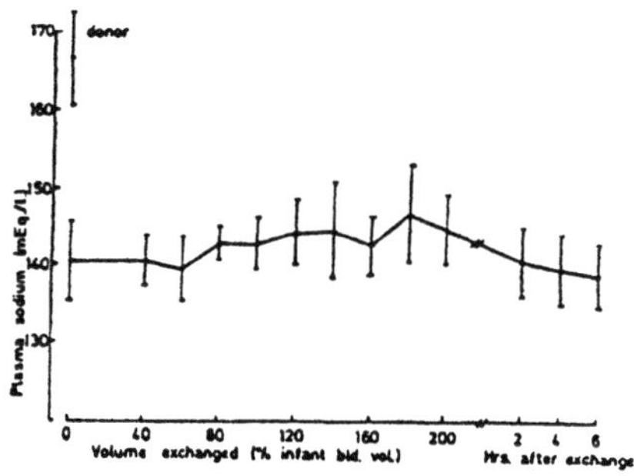

(from Tan and Tan 1975)[15]

Figure 2

PLASMA POTASSIUM LEVELS BEFORE, DURING AND AFTER EXCHANGE TRANSFUSION

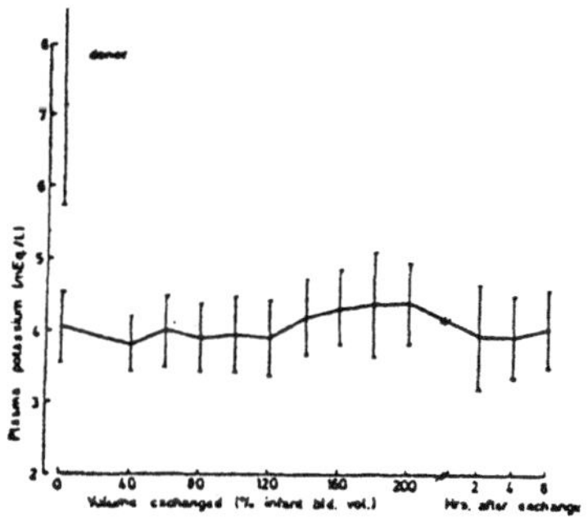

(From Tan and Tan 1975)[15]

deterioration may occur. The early anecdotal experience of exchange transfusion in both premature and full term infants attributed deterioration and death during exchange transfusion to hyperkalaemia and in more recent studies, infants < 1500 G demonstrated an excess of hypernatraemia in those who had an exchange transfusion, together with a higher incidence of germinal layer haemorrhage and intraventricular haemorrhage.[6]

There can thus be no doubt that hypernatraemia and hyperkalaemia subsequent to an exchange transfusion can cause problems in low birthweight short gestation infants.

Calcium

The fall in the level of this cation during exchange transfusion has been extensive studied, and Figs. 3, 4 and 5 from the paper by Maisels et al[9] summarise the data from their work and from the group in Toronto.[13] During exchange transfusion with ACD blood, partially due to the infusion of an ionised calcium free blood, and partially due to the chelation of the recipient's ionised calcium by the infused citrate, the level of ionised calcium in the recipient falls (Fig.3) though the total calcium remains the same or increases (Fig.4). Infusing calcium gluconate every 100 ml of exchange transfusion mitigates but does not prevent the fall in ionised calcium, but causes a rise in total plasma calcium. The effect of the calcium infusions is short lived (Fig.5).

Figure 3

SERUM IONISED CALCIUM IN INFANTS DURING EXCHANGE TRANSFUSION WITH HEPARINISED ACD BLOOD

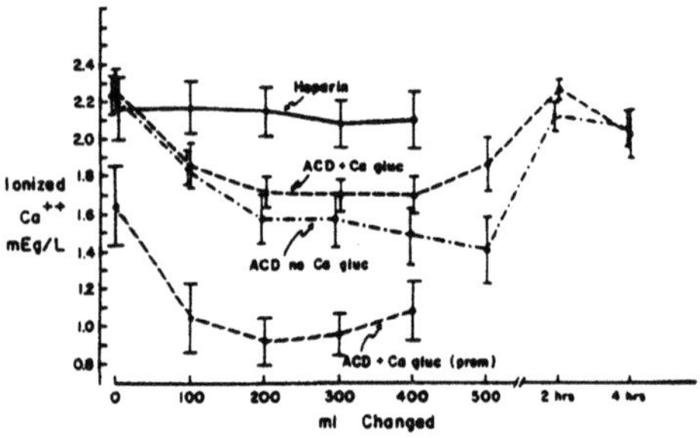

Infants receiving heparinised blood

Infants receiving 1 ml calcium gluconate every 100 ml exchange

Infants not receiving calcium gluconate

Term infants ± SEM

Preterm infants ± SEM

(from Maisels et al 1974)[9]

Figure 4

SERUM TOTAL CALCIUM IN INFANTS DURING EXCHANGE TRANSFUSION

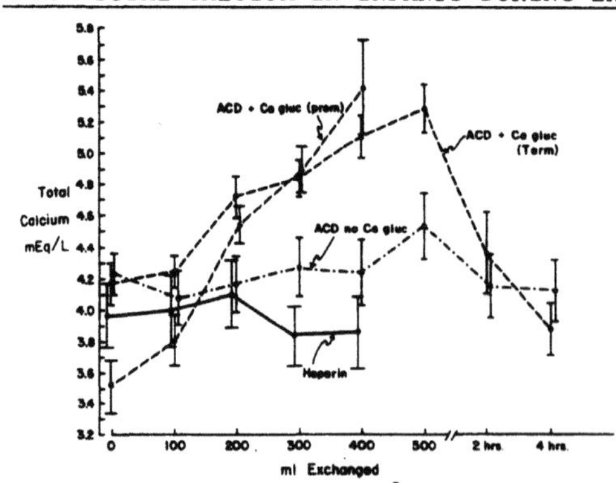

(From Maisels et al 1974)[9]

Figure 5

SERUM CONCENTRATIONS OF TOTAL AND IONISED CALCIUM

IMMEDIATELY BEFORE AND AFTER INFUSION OF 1 ml OF 10% CALCIUM GLUCONATE

DURING AN EXCHANGE TRANSFUSION WITH ACD BLOOD

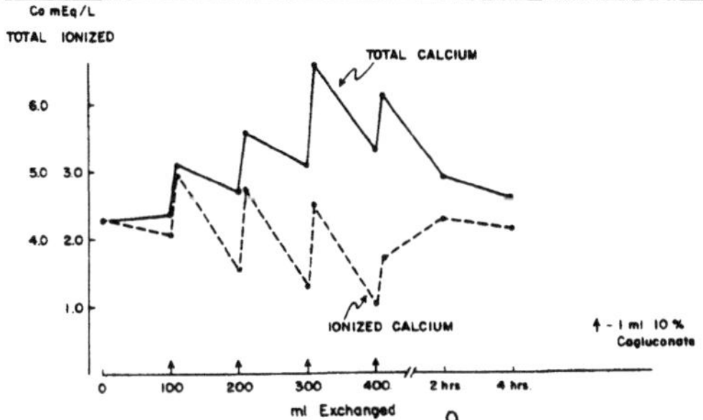

(from Maisels et al 1974)[9]

As might be expected the premature infant is more susceptible to these changes than a term infant, and a marked fall in plasma ionised calcium occurs in such infants (Fig.3). As Maisels et al[9] comment, it is surprising that more premature infants do not develop symptoms of hypocalcaemia during exchange transfusion. When they do, they rapidly respond to infusions of calcium gluconate (ideally given as 5 ml of 2% calcium gluconate) and in any case the ionised calcium values spontaneously return to normal within 10 minutes of stopping the infusion of citrates.

It is in the area of calcium homeostasis that the benefits of heparinised blood are most striking since in the absence of citrate, no changes in plasma calcium occur (Figs.3,4).

Acid Base Status

Acid citrate dextrose solution has a pH of 5.0 - 5.1, and citrate phosphate dextrose has a pH of 5.6 - 5.8. When these are added to a pint of blood they lower the pH to approximately 6.8 and approximately 7.15 respectively. In sealed containers the PCO_2 also rises to very high values (Table I). The pH of the stored blood gradually rises over the next three weeks, although over the first 3 - 4 days after collection it remains relatively constant.

Exchange transfusion with this acidaemic blood does cause a fall in the infant's pH, and an increase in his base deficit. The likelihood of metabolic acidaemia developing is much greater in infants exchange transfused on the first day of life.[4,8] In most cases the acidaemia is mild (Fig.6) and many experienced neonatologists assert that even then they never have any problem

Figure 6

PLASMA BICARBONATE DURING EXCHANGE TRANSFUSION WITH ACD BLOOD IN 14 MATURE BABIES

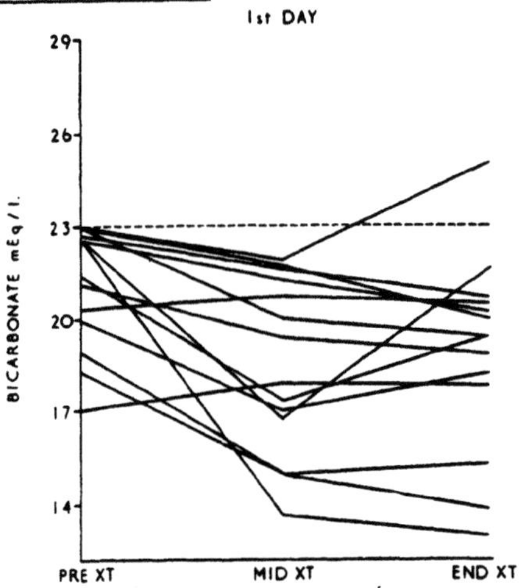

(from Calladine et al 1965)[4]

Figure 7

PCO_2 pH AND BICARBONATE IN A 2.00 kg BABY WHOSE CONDITION DETERIORATED DURING AN EXCHANGE TRANSFUSION WITH ACD BLO

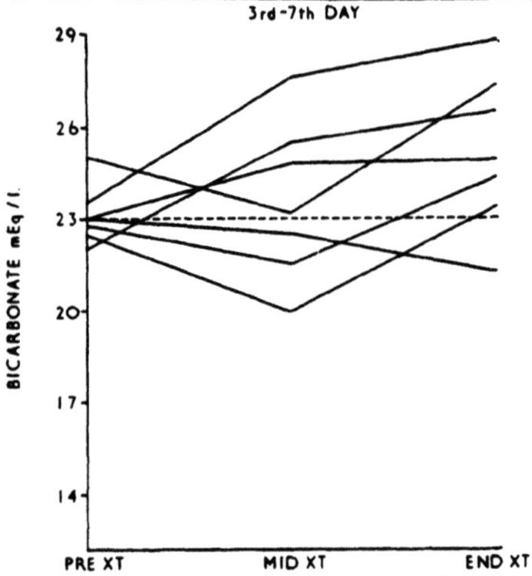

(from Calladine et al 1965)[4]

with acidaemia.[2] However, it is clear that in a few infants, particularly those of low birthweight who are already ill and acidotic before the exchange transfusion is started, profound, and potentially fatal acidaemia can develop (Fig.7).[8,12] For such infants ACD blood should have its pH corrected to about 7.0 - 7.1, using either bicarbonate or THAM,[7,11] since correction of the donor blood pH to > 7.0 - 7.1 results in a metabolic alkalaemia in the recipient 24 - 48 hours later. Whether CPD bloods needs correction of pH is an unanswered question, since it starts with a pH 0.2 - 0.3 points higher than ACD blood, (equivalent to 100 mEq/l(H)+), and at the pH level one is aiming to achieve when adding base to ACD blood. All the problems of metabolic acidaemia are of course avoided if fresh heparinised blood is used for the exchange transfusion.

2,3 Diphosphoglycerate (2,3 DPG)

A crucial component of the mechanism controlling the prime function of the RBC - the carriage of oxygen from the lungs, and its release to metabolically active cells, is the intracellular level of 2,3 DPG. An increase in this compound within the RBc decreases the affinity of haemoglobin for oxygen, thereby improving the release of oxygen to the tissues. A fall in intracellular 2,3 DPG

Figure 8

MEAN + - RANGES OF 2,3 DPG IN RED CELLS.

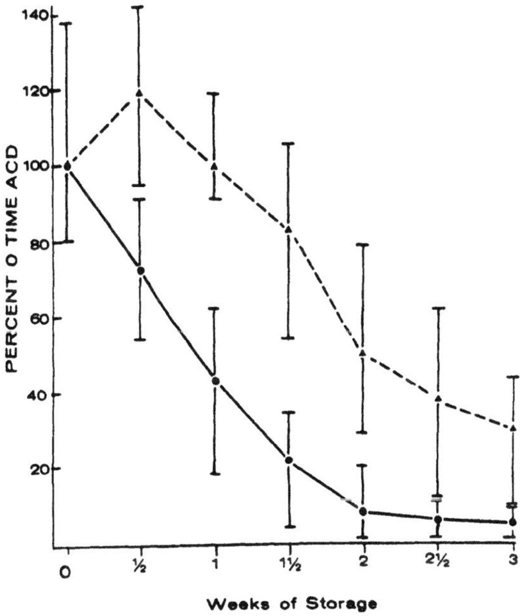

The 2,3 DPG level is given as the percentage activity compared with the original concentration in ACD blood (100%)

-- ▲ -- CPD blood

— ● — ACD blood

(from Shafer et al 1971)[14]

has the reverse effect, tending to hold oxygen on to the haemoglobin and compromise tissue oxygenation. It is therefore crucial that the level of 2,3 DPG is sustained in bank blood. Figure 8 shows that it is very much better maintained in CPD blood than ACD blood.

The oxygen affinity of blood (measured as the P_{50}) is also affected by the fetal haemoglobin level - which reduces oxygen release and the P_{50}, and acute acidaemia which increases the oxygen release and P_{50}.

Bearing all these variables in mind, the effect in exchange transfusion in infants with < 24 hour old or 4 - 5 day old ACD blood containing primary adult

Figure 9

P_{50}(solid line), TOTAL 2:3 DPG (open histogram)
AND FUNCTIONING DPG FRACTION (total 2,3 DPG x % HbA - shaded histogram)
IN INFANTS BEFORE AND AFTER EXCHANGE TRANSFUSION
WITH <24 HOUR OLD OR 4-5 DAY OLD ACD BLOOD

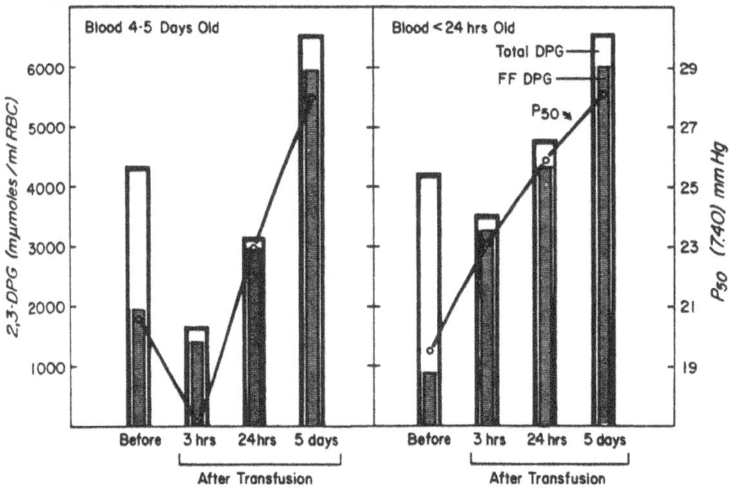

(from Delivoria-Papadopoulos et al 1971)[5]

haemoglobin is shown in Figure 9. With < 24 hour blood, despite the slight fall in 2:3 DPG caused by transfusing low 2,3 DPG blood the substitution of the infant's fetal haemoglobin with the donor's adult haemoglobin which interacts better with 2,3 DPG raises the recipient's P_{50}, and this improvement continues on subsequent days as the 2,3 DPG regenerates within the transfused RBC. Using 4 - 5 day old blood the results are very different. Immediately after the exchange transfusion there is a marked fall in P_{50} which, even though it recovers within 24 hours, could, in the immediate post-exchange transfusion period, further compromise tissue oxygenation in a sick infant.[5]

Bursaux et al[3] have shown that similar deleterious changes occur with 2 day old ACD blood. Their data also clearly demonstrates the superiority of CPD blood < 2 days old. When this is used for exchange transfusion there is an immediate increase in the P_{50} of the infant's blood following exchange transfusion. Heparinised blood would also be expected to cause an instant rise in the infant's P_{50} following exchange transfusion, since it too substitutes adult low affinity for fetal high affinity haemoglobin.

Conclusion

It can be seen that for the three factors discussed, exchange transfusion causes major biochemical and physiological changes. These are particularly severe when using ACD blood, less when using CPD blood, and unlikely when using heparinised blood. Whichever type of donor blood is used, the severity of the metabolic changes is greater the older the blood.

Acknowledgements

My thanks are due to my secretary Miss Janita Whittingham for typing this manuscript.

REFERENCES

1. Bolande R.P., Traisman, H.S. and H.F. Philipsborn: Electrolyte considerations in exchange transfusion for erythroblastosis fetalis. J.Pediat. 49:401, 1956.

2. Bowman, J.M.: Neonatal Management. In: Modern Management of the Rhesus Problem by J.T. Queenan, Medical Department Harper & Tow, 1977, p. 215.

3. Bursaux, E., Freminet, A., Brossard, Y. and C.F. Poyart: Exchange transfusion in the neonate with ACD or CPD stored blood. Biology of the Neonate, 23:123, 1973.

4. Calladine, M., Gairdner, D., Maidoo, B.T. and D.H. Orrell: Acid base changes following exchange transfusion with citrated blood. Arch.Dis.Child. 40:626, 1965.

5. Delivoria-Papadopoulos, M., Morrow, G., and F.A. Oski: Exchange transfusion in the newborn infant with fresh and old blood. The role of storage on 2:3 diphosphoglycerate, haemoglobin oxygen affinity and oxygen release. J.Pediat. 79:898, 1971.

6. Doyle, E., Eidelman A.I., Lee, K.S., Daum, C. and L.M. Gartner: Exchange transfusion and hypernatraemia: possible role in intracranial haemorrhage in very low birthweight infants. J.Pediat. 92:848, 1978.

7. Gandy, G.M., Partridge, J.W. and D. Gairdner: Control of acidosis during exchange transfusion with citrate blood. Arch.Dis. Child. 43:147, 1968.

8. Hervei, S., Malik, T., and M. Rotfaluzy: Acid base changes of mature and premature neonates following exchange transfusion. Biology of the Neonate, 29:323, 1976.

9. Maisels, M.J., Li, T.K., Piechocki, J.T., and M.V. Werthman: The effect of exchange transfusion on serum ionised calcium. Pediatrics 53:683, 1974.

10. Miller, G., McCoord, A.B., Joos, H.A., and S.W. Clausen: Studies on serum electrolyte changes during exchange transfusion. Pediatrics 13:412, 1954.

11. Person, W.E., Barrett, C.T.and T.K. Oliver: The effect of buffered and non-buffered ACD blood on electrolyte and acid base homeostasis during exchange transfusion. Pediatrics 41:802, 1968.

12. Povey, M.J.C.: pH changes during exchange transfusion. Lancet ii:339, 1964.

13. Radde, I.C., Parkinson, D.K., Hoffen, B., Appiah, K.E. and W.B. Hanley: Calcium ion activity in the sick neonate: Effect of bicarbonate administration and exchange transfusion. Ped.Res.6:43, 1972.

14. Shafer, A.W., Tague, L.L., Welch, M.H. and C.A. Guenter: 2:3 DPG in red cells stored in ACD and CPD. Implications regarding delivery of oxygen. J.Lab.clin.Med. 77:430, 1971.

15. Tan, K.L. and I.K. Tan: Plasma potassium, sodium and chloride levels during and after exchange transfusion. Aust.Paediat.J. 11:165, 1975.

----

4. EXCHANGE TRANSFUSION: METABOLIC ASPECTS AND BIOCHEMICAL CHANGES

A.S. KHALIFA

The incidence of haemolytic disease of the newborn due to Rhesus incompatibility has been markedly reduced since the introduction of Rhesus isoimmunisation prophylaxis. Anti-D immunoglobulin is given to all Rhesus (D) negative women without antibodies during delivery of a Rhesus (D) positive baby (liveborn, stillborn or abortion after the 20th week). This is regardless of the parity of the patient or of the ABO group of the baby. A failure of 1.6% of this prophylaxis initiated the need for anti-D immunoglobulin administration to all D-negative women at 28 weeks of gestational age.[13]

Exchange transfusion is still life saving in a group of clinico-pathological states:-

1. Hyperbilirubinaemia due to different causes (Table I) is one of the most important indications for exchange transfusion.

TABLE I

	Rh.	ABO	L.B. wt	G6PD def	Vit K	Ex. Haematoma	Toxo	?
Total	49	15	8	4	4	3	2	5
Males	32	8	5	4	2	2	1	3
Females	17	7	3	-	2	1	1	2

2. As a detoxifying measure exchange transfusion is indicated and is of value. Children are exposed to a group of drugs which may remain in the circulation for some time, or drugs which are highly protein bound or are closely associated with cellular elements in the blood. These drugs include antihistamine, diphenoxylate, barbiturates and cyanides. Cyanides are to be found in bitter almond oil and as a by product of the amygdaline ingested from apple seeds or unripe gawafa or olives and

changed to cyanides by stomach acidity and body temperature. Exchange transfusion is especially helpful in small children in whom the technical difficulties of haemodialysis are great.[9,12]

3. In Reye Syndrome exchange transfusion might be life saving in severe stages III and IV with severe encephalopathy, severe hyper-ammoniaemia and marked coagulation defects. Coagulation defects in Reye Syndrome have been attributed to decreased production of all coagulation factors except Factor VIII. However, consumption coagulopathy was also confirmed.[4]
4. Exchange transfusion is the most efficient method of decreasing the number of sickle cells in sickle cell anaemia to treat vaso-occlusive crises and in preparing such patients for surgery. The percentage of haemoglobin-S should be reduced to below 30%. This technique can be supplemented by a continuous programme in which red blood cells are given every 3 - 4 weeks. The aim of this therapy is the suppression of erythropoiesis, so eliminating the production of sickle cells.[8]
5. Exchange transfusion was reported by Delivoria et al in 1971,[3] 1974,[1] and 1976[2] as significantly increasing survival in respiratory distress syndrome. Adult haemoglobin given to the newly born has higher 2,3 diphosphoglycerate and a relatively right-shifted oxygen dissociation curve than fetal haemoglobin leading to a better tissue oxygenation.

Hypoglycaemia associated with haemolytic disease of the newborn, particularly severe cases, was described by Price in 1969.[11] Dextrose is required to prevent brain damage and is also necessary in the conjugation of bilirubin. Hyperinsulinism was confirmed in the plasma of infants with HDN due to Rh immunisation by Mølsted-Pederson et al in 1973.[10]

The metabolic risks of exchange transfusion include hyperkalaemia, hypocalcaemia, hypomagnesaemia, acidosis, hypoglycaemia and hypernatraemia. This paper reports on exchange transfusions administered to more than 90 newborns with hyperbilirubinaemia whose aetiologies are shown in Table I. Acid Citrate Dextrose (ACD) treated blood was used in preference to heparinised blood since the latter cannot be stored for more than 24 hours and causes a rise in plasma concentration of NEFA that competes with bilirubin for albumin binding sites. Human serum albumin in 20% solution was given in a dose of 1 g/Kg body- weight for 10 patients before exchange and one volume exchange was done. The dose of albumin was repeated. The infant was left for 1 hour to give ample time for the albumin to bind the circulating bilirubin. Thereafter a second volume exchange transfusion was completed.

TABLE II

	Serum-Bilirubin Before Exch.	After Exch.	Post-Exch. %
No HSA	25.7 ± 5.2	15.2 ± 2	59± 5
With HSA	19.9 ± 3	9.1 ± 1.5	45 ± 4

P:< 0.01

Table II presents the pre- and post-exchange bilirubin levels in patients receiving human serum albumin infusions as compared to those not receiving the albumin. It is clear that the albumin infusion increases significantly the efficiency of exchange transfusion as detected by the post-exchange percentage. Not only that, but none of the patients receiving the human serum albumin required a second exchange. On the other hand, 25% of the other patients required one or more exchanges. It has been demonstrated that intravenous administration of albumin prior to exchange transfusion results in decreased serum bilirubin concentration due to binding of mobilised bilirubin and increased effectiveness of the process. As much as 30% or 40% more bilirubin can be removed in this way. Since the addition of albumin in the blood expands the blood volume, it should not be used in severe anaemia with increased blood volume or in cases of cardiac failure.[5]

The pre- and post-exchange levels of bilirubin, serum glutamic oxalacetic transaminase, serum sodium and potassium are presented in Tables IV and V. Table III presents the normal range. It is clear that in acute haemolysis, the hyperbilirubinaemia is associated with elevated levels of SGOT. This enzyme, being almost exclusively confined within the cells like other intracellular enzymes, enters the extracellular phase of body fluids in small amounts as a result of the normal wear and tear of the cells. In cases of haemolysis,

TABLE III

	Bilirubin (mg %)	SGOT (units)	Na(mEq/L)	K(mEq/L)
Normal				
Range	0.5 - 1	3 - 14	134 - 150	3.55 - 6.7
Mean	0.8	8.2	140.5	4.2
S.D. ±	0.2	5	4.2	0.6

TABLE IV

Rh INCOMPATIBILITY

	Bilirubin (mg%)	SGOT (units)	Na (mEq/L)	K (mEq/L)	Hgb (gms%)
Before Exchange					
Range	10.2 - 39	14 - 30	120 - 160	3.9 - 7	10 - 14
Mean	7.1	23	140.5	5.28	12
S.D. ±	8.4	5.8	12.6	0.87	1.2
P	< 0.001	< 0.001	Insign.	< 0.01	
After Exchange					
Range	6 - 22	4.7 - 20.5	125 - 100	2.7 - 4.8	
Mean	13.7	12	142.2	3.89	
S.D. ±	4.7	4.6	12	0.76	
P	< 0.001	Insign.	Insign.	Insign.	

P: between normal and each of the groups.

increased permeability of even actual damage of the cells allows intracellular enzymes to escape at a greater rate. The rise of SGOT in the patients with congenital toxoplasmosis was more marked. This might be explained by the more extensive damage where gross necrosis occurs in many tissues, especially the heart, lungs, skeletal muscles, liver, spleen and the nervous system.

TABLE V

A B O

	Bilirubin (mg%)	SGOT (units)	Na (mEq/L)	K (mEq/L)	Hgb (gms%)
Before Exchange					
Range	21.5-25.4	14 - 20	135 - 145	4.1 - 6.5	12 - 15
Mean	22.6	17	139	5.12	12.8
S.D. ±	2.4	3	5.4	0.78	2
P	< 0.001	< 0.001	Insign.	< 0.01	
After Exchange					
Range	5.6 -15.2	4.5 - 8	132.6-155	3.2 - 6.5	
Mean	11.1	6.8	140	4.5	
S.D. ±	4.1	2.4	7.5	1.42	
P	< 0.001	Insign.	Insign.	Insign.	

The rise in serum potassium in the haemolytic process can be explained by destruction of cells with liberation of potassium from the cells and also as a manifestation of stress. This increase in serum potassium will necessitate using fresh blood for transfusion in haemolytic processes to avoid potassium toxicity. The serum sodium, however, was within normal levels except in the two patients with toxoplasmosis (Table VI). These patients manifested evidence of heart

TABLE VI

CASES OF CONGENITAL TOXOPLASMOSIS

	Bilirubin (mg%)	SGOT (units)	Na (mEq/L)	K (mEq/L)
Case 1:	18	120	150	7.5
	12	80	130	5
Case 2:	14.5	105	160	6
	8	20.5	142.5	4.2

failure. After exchange, the sodium level returned to within normal levels.[6] Our experience in Reye Syndrome[7] comprises 7 children with Grades III and IV encephalopathy. Five were females and 2 males, aged from 2 - 12 years. Patients were subjected to quick prothrombin time (PT), partial thromboplastin time (PTT), thrombin time (TT), and platelet count. Assay of Factors I (fibrinogen), II, V, VII, VIII and IX was determined. Serum fibrin(ogen) degradation products (FDP) were measured by the staphyloccal clumping test. These tests were done on admission, 24, 48 and 72 hours later. Patients received 2-volume exchange transfusion. Peritoneal or haemodialysis was undertaken if the BUN was rising, in the presence of electrolyte disturbance and/or deteriorating sensorium and clinical conditions. Platelets were reduced in 1 patient, fibrinogen decreased in 4, and FDP was positive in 5. Factor II level was depressed in 2, Factor V in all patients, Factor VII in 4 and Factors VIII and IX in 3. PTT was particularly increased. After 24 hours and the 2-volume exchange transfusion, the coagulation tests remained the same or had even deteriorated. At 48 hours the platelet count was low in 4 patients and fibrinogen levels decreased. Factor V levels were decreased and these children expired. In the remaining 3 children the general condition improved, although at 72 hours the coagulation parameters were still abnormal. These children survived although 2 of them manifested neuromuscular problems that necessitated rehabilitation and physiotherapy. These findings could reflect an imbalance of hepatic production, fibrinolytic activators and inhibitors or lack of clearance by the RES. An added element of DIC may be functioning as evidenced by thrombocytopenia, low levels of Factor VIII and lack of correction of clotting factor deficiency following fresh frozen plasma infusion, exchange transfusion and renal dialysis.

Conclusions

Some of the biochemical changes presented could be considered as criteria of severity of the haemolytic process and their return to normal provides laboratory data for the efficiency of exchange transfusion. ACD is of value as an anticoagulant to prevent hypoglycaemia provided calcium is given in the dose of 1 ml per 100 ml exchanged to prevent hypocalcaemia. The use of human serum albumin before exchange and after one volume exchange was found to be of significant value in helping to reduce the bilirubin level and to obviate a second exchange.

Exchange is a life saving measure in certain toxicities, particularly cyanides, together with such other measures as methylene blue or thiosulphate injections. In severe types of Reye Syndrome, exchange transfusion failed to normalise the coagulation defects present, but it is still indicated to get rid of hyper-ammonaemia and to correct a high BUN, together with other treatment measures.

TABLE VII

COAGULATION TESTS IN REYE SYNDROME

Patient	Age in years	Sex	Time of test	Platelets	PT	PTT	TT	Fibrinogen	FDP	Factors II	V	VII	VIII	IX	Remarks
1) SR	7 2/12	W/F	0	N	+	++	N	N	+	-	-	--	-	-	Expired
			72 hrs	-	+	++	++	-	++	--	--	--	--	-	
2) AC	6	W/F	0	N	N	N	N	-	++	N	--	N	N	N	Expired
3) SV	9	B/F	0	N	N	+	N	-	++	N	--	-	N	N	Expired
			72 hrs	-	+	++	+			-	--	-	-	-	
4) PD	12	W/M	0	N	+	+	N	-	++	N	--	-	-	-	Expired
			72 hrs	-	+	+	+	-	++	N	--	-	-	-	
5) WV	8	W/F	0	N	N	+	N	N	neg	N	-	-	-	-	
			72 hrs	-	N	N	N	N	neg	N	-	-	N	-	
6) DH	2	W/M	0	N	N	+	N	N	neg	-	--	N	N	N	
			72 hrs	N	N	N	N	N	neg	N	-	N	N	N	
7) LM	2	W/F	0	-	N	+	N	N	++	N	--	N	N	N	
			72 hrs	--	N	+	+	-	+	N	-	N	N	N	

N = within normal range
+ = abnormally prolonged or elevated
- = abnormally low

REFERENCES

1. Delivoria-Papadopoulos, M., Martens, M., Roncevic, N.P. and F.A. Oski: Postnatal changes in oxygen transport of term and sick infants. The role of red cell 2,3 diphosphoglycerate and adult haemoglobin. Pediat.Res. 5:235, 1974.

2. Delivoria-Papadopoulos M., Miller, L.D., and R.E. Forester: The role of exchange transfusion in the management of low birthweight infants with or without respiratory distress syndrome. J.Pediat. 89:273, 1976.

3. Delivoria-Papadopoulos M., Morrow, G., and F.A. Oski: Exchange transfusion in the newborn with fresh and old blood, effects on oxygen release. J.Pediat. 78:879, 1971.

4. Hilby, M.D., McClung, H.J., Haynes, R.E., Romsche, C.A. and E.S. Sharad: Reye Syndrome in siblings. J.Pediat. 94:576, 1979.

5. Khalifa, A.S., and K.A.H. Mourad: Clinical experience in the management of icterus gravis neonatorum. Ains Shams med.J. 23:477, 1972.

6. Khalifa, A.S., Mourad, K.A.H. and S. Eid: Correlation between severity of the haemolytic process and some biochemical changes in acute haemolysis. J.Egypt.Med.Assoc. 56:407, 1973.

7. Kosmidis, H.V., Khalifa, A.S., Arcinue, E., Sarnaik, A., Adelman,S., and J.M. Lusher: Coagulation abnormalities in Reye Syndrome. (in press), 1980.

8. Lusher, J.M., Haghight, H. and A.S. Khalifa: A prophylactic transfusion program for children with sickle cell anemia complicated by CNS infarction. Am.J.Hematol. 1:265, 1976.

9. Teitelbaum, D.T., and L.C. Kier: Arsine poisoning. Arch.environ.Hlth. 19:133, 1969.

10. Mølsted-Pederson, L., Trautner, H., and K.R. Jørgensen: Plasma insulin and K values during intravenous glucose tolerance test in newborn infants with erythroblastosis fetalis. Acta paediat.Scand. 62:11, 1973.

11. Price, H.V.: Hypoglycaemia complicating haemolytic disease of the newborn. Arch.Dis.Childh. 44:248, 1969.

12. Mann, J.B. and D.H. Sandberg: Therapy of sedative overdosage. Pediat.Clin.N.Amer. 17:617, 1970.

13. Tovey, L.A.D.: Failures of prevention of Rh immunisation: causes and consequences. Joint meeting, 18th Congress, Intl.Soc.Hematology and 16th Congress, Intl.Soc. Blood Transfusion, Montreal, Canada,1980.

5. DISCUSSION

moderator: S.P. ISRAËLS

Dudok DE WIT (Den Haag, Netherlands): Professor Forfar's wide ranging review of Rhesus disease left out one aspect - something that has haunted me personally for some fifteen years. One of my own first patients with Rhesus antibodies and with complications, including anti-C, had a very high bilirubin. I had expected that an exchange transfusion would be carried out. But, the hospital - a university children's hospital - advised that it was their practice to look only at the bilirubin. In this instance it was not indirect and not dangerous and they would not do an exchange transfusion for this child.

However, the concern in the literature was always with bilirubin and the distinction is never made.

J.O.FORFAR: In speaking of hyperbilirubinaemia in the context of haemolytic disease of the newborn I was speaking only of indirect-acting bilirubin. In practice - not wholly but to a very large extent - we discount direct-acting bilirubin as having a different significance altogether in terms of the unlikely effect that it will have in causing any brain damage, unlike the indirect acting, which will produce brain damage. Any interest in direct-acting bilirubin has a totally different connotation. We have some interest in this in terms of hepatic function but not in terms of the brain damage that we are discussing and the sequelae of HDN.

A.S. KHALIFA: I acknowledge the bravery and courage of Dr. Turner in showing us his results. For example, in his figures on treatment, although the treatment was efficient as regards the coagulation studies done the mortality rate was still 76.2%.

One question: what is the reptilase time? What does it indicate and how is it done?

Th.L. TURNER: Reptilase time is a qualitative measure of fibrinogen. Dr Khalifa will have to look up the literature as I have to; I cannot tell him offhand how it is done. There are commercial reagents available for reptilase time.

L.S. DE VRIES (Utrecht, Netherlands): In Amsterdam they are currently doing a study on antithrombin-III, the main inhibitor of thrombin for the coagulation system. It is said that in the newborn it is a bit low, lower than in adults, and in premature infants it is very low. They say that if a child is suspected of having a DIC, heparin will only function if there is enough antithrombin in the system, and they suggest that it may be better to give the child fresh frozen plasma containing antithrombin-III, in combination with heparin. Does Dr. Turner have any experience with antithrombin-III?

T.L. TURNER: I have no direct experience with it but I have experience of using the three products, cryoprecipitate, prothrombin complex and platelet with heparin. It did not make management of those infants with severe DIC in the newborn period either significantly easier or more difficult.

A. OKKEN (Groningen, Netherlands): In his presentation, Dr Roberton put the metabolic effects of an exchange transfusion, whether with ACD, CPD or heparinised blood into a perspective of gestational age, birthweight and age of the infant. I believe that to be very important. As a neonatologist, I would be very interested in his suggestions as to the future of exchange transfusions in small babies as we might in due course be using either other anticoagulants or different compositions of exchange blood. What would Dr. Roberton suggest we use or look for in the next few years?

N.R.C. ROBERTON: In babies under 1500 gms or 1700 gms, the fresher the blood the better. Even 2-day old or 3-day old blood in those babies can in a percentage, if they start sick, cause metabolic deterioration. We also have to look at why the baby is to be exchanged, and in quite a few instances the baby will have sepsis, or DIC on its own, or sepsis plus DIC. In that situation there is a great deal to be said for having heparinised blood - theoretically. I have not used heparinised blood for a long time. In Cambridge we use CPD blood. When I did use heparinised blood at Hammersmith and at Oxford there was no doubt that the babies did extremely well - the very small babies - when they were exchanged with it, and that they had minimal complications from it.

Perhaps the message I would give is that somebody who has a huge experience of exchanging small babies - we do not have a large one; we draw the prems from about 10,000 deliveries a year and that does not give us a huge experience - somebody that can draw on 40,000 deliveries a year, eg, Cooke County, Chicago, or Toronto, Canada, should look at what happens during exchange with CPD blood. I think ACD blood is a disaster with such small babies but someone with sufficient data to draw on should look at the experience with CPD blood and monitor, as the Tans* and Professor Khalifa** have done, carefully during the exchange transfusion and actually see what happens. I do not think the data yet exists on which anyone can base a good critique of CPD blood against heparinised blood.

A.S. KHALIFA: In fact we must take a careful look at the role of heparin in treating DIC conditions. Five years ago everybody was trying to use heparin for everything: in haemolytic uraemic syndrome, in DIC and in everything. But now, in the literature, we can find that there is a lot of doubt about the efficiency of heparin in the control of these conditions.

P.C. DAS (Groningen, Netherlands): In Scotland almost all the blood supplied will be CPD. I left Scotland in 1977 and for the previous three years no heparinised blood had been supplied in Edinburgh. The only clinical condition I know of where we used to supply it was that of "groggy babies", to use Scottish terminology, ie, the preterm babies with DIC or infection. Dr. Roberton has told us that in England he uses CPD blood. In Groningen we have supplied CPD blood since 1976. Dr. Kerr told of a case where a baby was born in Glasgow suddenly without planned exchange transfusion and she used the blood that was ready and available, and to which her registrar had access, to save that baby's life. I am not clear what Dr. Turner or Dr. Roberton would do in that situation, ie, in an emergency by contrast to the planned exercise. Perhaps Dr. Kerr could tell us exactly what she did when this case arrived on her doorstep and clarify the position.

M.M. KERR (Glasgow, Scotland): We insist that such blood should always be available in any maternity hospital. Almost always it will be needed for the mother. Very occasionally, perhaps once a year, it will be needed for the babies. This is what our haematologists call screened O-negative CPD blood. It is extremely precious merely because it is so time-consuming to produce. It keeps being renewed. We are not supposed to use it except in a case of dire emergency. It is kept in the labour suite, not even in the haematology department, and it is available for any mother who is literally bleeding to death, as perinatal patients can, or for her baby in a similar situation; the exsanguinated baby at birth. We have had this practice for many years in our

*Tan, K.L. and I.K. Tan: Aust.Paediat.J. 11:165, 1975.
**Khalifa, A.S.: Proceedings, 5th Annual Bloodbank Symposium, Groningen,1981.

maternity hospital and it should be common practice in any maternity hospital worth the name.

Screened O-negative blood is blood that is known not to contain any antibody as far as modern testing can discover. It is always available.

J.O.FORFAR: Despite what Dr. Das has said, we do use heparinised blood in Edinburgh but we use heparinised citrated blood. It is used in bypass surgery, which is being increasingly applied to babies of very low birthweight. There is not the slightest doubt that they get very high citrate levels, much higher than we get in our exchange transfusion babies, and in following them up, as far as we can make out they tolerate these citrate levels very well, at least in the short term, although we do not have the long-term follow ups that have been discussed.

J. VAN HALLE (Keekbergen, Belgium): Could Dr. Roberton comment about the possible adverse effects of citrate per se independent of the calcium effect?

N.R.C. ROBERTON: Not with ease, no. I struggle slightly with citrate metabolism. There is quite a bit in the literature that implies that in addition to chelating calcium, and that poisonous effect of citrate, very high plasma citrate levels, 100 mgs percent or above, are in themselves toxic. I am not quite clear how they are supposed to be toxic but they are supposed to be toxic. But my reading of the literature is that a lot of acid citrate blood would have to be given very quickly to get that sort of plasma level and for it to have any effect on the baby. The sort of effect it will have on the baby is that the baby will just "go off" a bit. It will go a bit acidaemic and a bit hypertensive. All the other things that I have talked about today can have that same effect and it is very difficult to separate out from what goes wrong during an exchange transfusion to make the baby hypotensive and "groggy" into individual components of the blood being given to it.

The other effect is that it is metabolised eventually to bicarbonate and the baby can become alkalaemic. In Cambridge, 10 - 15 years ago, when they looked at this methodically they found that if they tried to correct the pH of ACD blood too much towards normal, then the baby could become very alkalaemic with a pH of 7.55 and bicarb of 35 two days later. The babies did not seem to come to much harm on it, but nevertheless their metabolic boots were not clean. But I do not think that the evidence is clear exactly as to what citrate does or whether it is very poisonous.

C.Th. SMIT SIBINGA (Groningen, Netherlands): In 1950, thirty years ago, Mollison and Veall* suggested that if any problem was to be expected on the metabolic side, especially on donor blood for exchange transfusion in haemolytic disease of the newborn, half of the plasma should be taken out and the exchange done with a unit of what Mollison** called modified whole blood. That is red cells together with half of the plasma volume, providing a unit of blood with a haematocrit which is far more adequate for a neonate than a normal standard adult unit of blood.

Secondly, I recently came across some information provided by Kevy*** of the children's hospital medical school in Boston. They are converting regular CPD blood, 2 - 5 days old into heparin blood by adding heparin and calcium gluconate. Kevy says that in these cases technically the exchange transfusions "run a bit more smoothly" because of not having to add calcium and doing the exchange at the same time with the same pair of hands. If the citrate is regarded as inconvenient to the newborn, especially the premature, it would be very simple to remove half the plasma and lower the loadings of citrate, sodium and potassium. Both products, modified whole blood and heparin converted CPD blood, can be made available off the shelf. Screened and quality controlled blood is there for immediate and safe use!

----

*Veall and Mollison, P.L.: Lancet, 2:792, 1950.
**Mollison, P.L.: Blood transfusion in clinical medicine, 6th ed., Blackwell Scientific Publications, Oxford, 1979.
***Kevy, S.V.: Paediatric Transfusion Therapy. In: Transfusion Therapy, A.A.B.B., Washington, 1974.
Kevy, S.V.: Personal Communication, 1 December 1976.
Kevy, S.V.: Personal Communication, 30 September 1980.

1. PAEDIATRICS AND BLOODTRANSFUSION: PRACTICAL ASPECTS

J.O. FORFAR

INTRODUCTION

Blood is a remarkable fluid. It has been available from time immemorial but we have only learnt in recent times of its possible value as a therapy and even more recently of how to use it effectively in treatment. Whatever the colour of a man's skin, the colour of his blood is the same. To my knowledge there is no scientific support for the reputed 'blue blood' which the aristocracy of England are supposed to posses.

Practical aspects of blood usage must take account of the many properties which blood possesses. It is fluid but clots under certain circumstances: it is under constant movement as it circulates round the body: within the vascular system it maintains a pressure normally within certain clearly defined limits: its temperature is maintained within a narrow range: it has a complex composition maintaining a number of different formed elements in a fluid matrix: it has a wide range of immunological and anti-infective properties: all the elements have important chemical and metabolic functions not only per se but in an interreacting manner with each other.

BLOOD AND BLOOD PRODUCTS

A few may still remember the situation where blood was looked upon as a single entity and transfusion consisted of removing blood from a donor, collecting it into a bottle with citrate in it and promptly transfusing the waiting recipient. Today there is a considerable array of different blood preparations and blood products. These are shown in Table I, subdivided into whole blood, formed elements and plasma products.

In the use of blood and blood products the paediatrician has to go beyond the simple concept of replacing blood lost or destroyed. He has to come to terms with antigens and antibodies of increasing complexity and esoteric designation, immunoglobulins and immune responses, T cells and labelled cells, HLA types and blood group types and a galaxy of coagulation factors. Blood is

TABLE I

A STORED BLOOD - WHOLE

Type	Comment
Heparinised	Tends to clot, short storage (60% rbc survival 6-10 days), free fatty acid effect, heparinisation risk
Acid-citrate-dextrose (ACD)	80% rbc survival at 21 days: electrolyte effects
Citrate-phosphate-dextrose (CPD)	80% rbc survival at 32 days: electrolyte effects
Citrate-phospate-dextrose + adenine	Longer rbc survival especially after 3 wks storage: electrolyte effects

B BLOOD PRODUCTS - FORMED ELEMENTS

Packed cells/red cell suspensions	Higher Hb conc.: less disturb. blood volume: plasma saved
Washed red cells	Less antigenic stim. and transfusion reaction: v. short life: possible contamination
Platelet suspension	Thrombocytopenia: qualitative defects of platelets
Separated leucocytes	Infected neutropenic subjects

C BLOOD PRODUCTS - PLASMA AND ITS DERIVATIVES

Fresh plasma/fresh frozen plasma/dried plasma	Volume restoration; burns; hypoalbuminaemia; Factor VIII and IX deficiencies
Purified protein fraction (PPF)	Hypoalbuminaemia; oligaemia
Albumin (purified; salt poor)	Hypoalbuminaemia; neonatal jaundice; oligaemia
Cryoprecipitate	Coagulation defects involving Factors I and VIII
Prothrombin complex (four factor concentrate)	Coagulation defects involving Factors II, VII, IX, X
Immunoglobulin	Hypogammaglobulinaemia;infective hepatitis; rubella; measles
Rh anti-D Ig	Prevention of HDN due to Rh incompatibility

no longer a single homogeneous substance: it can be whole, its red cells can be packed and washed. The cell separator puts the individual formed elements of blood, red cells, white cells and platelets at the disposal of the clinician and can also, of course, remove from the patient certain elements of blood which may be unwanted. Plasma is no longer merely blood from which the cells have been removed: it can be obtained fresh, dried or fresh frozen: it can be fractionated to produce therapeutic substances such as cryoprecipitate and prothrombin complex (4 factor concentrate). The clinician may not fully understand the basic science which has gone into these developments but has to try and obtain a working knowledge of their implications in clinical practice, of how blood and blood products can best be used and of how they can be used most effectively and efficiently, bearing in mind their scarcity. We have an obligation to make the best possible use of the resources of blood transfusion services in view of the important personal contribution made by blood donors and the cost of the services in terms of personnel, accommodation and equipment.

TABLE II

HEPARINISED BLOOD

Pro	Con
Better preservation of platelets and granulocytes	Has to be freshly obtained
No citrate effect	Anticoagulant effect
No acidotic effect	Clots tend to occur
No hyper/hypo-glycaemic effect	Raises free fatty acids
No sodium load	Higher rate of infection
	Waste and expense

CITRATED BLOOD

Pro	Con
More readily available	Citrate effect
No heparin effect	Acidotic
No clotting	Hyper/hypo-glycaemic effect
No free fatty acid effect	Sodium load
Less risk of infection	Platelets and granulocytes less viable

There is some controversy on the relative merits of citrated and heparinised blood, a controversy which is particularly relevant to paediatrics. Table II summarises the arguments. There are many theoretical factors in blood transfusion and the protagonists of one type of preserved blood can always find arguments to support their views. In Edinburgh, and indeed in Britain, the balance of advantage at all ages is seen to lie with citrated blood. In the context of paediatrics the factors that have led to a judgement in favour of citrated blood are shown in Table II.

The degrees of hyper- and hypoglycaemia resulting from the use of citrate/ dextrose blood are not marked, ranging from a high of 180 mg per cent (10.0 mmol/l) to a low of 20 mg per cent (1.1 mmol/l).[6] These are unlikely to have much adverse effect and if need be can be readily controlled by insulin and glucose.

The plasma sodium concentration in citrated blood is of the order of 322 mg/dl or 168 mmol/l. Simmons et al (1974)[8] drew attention to the possibility that the treatment of acidosis with sodium bicarbonate in the newborn infant might be a cause of intraventricular haemorrhage. This conclusion was subsequently disputed by Anderson et al.[1] On the basis of Simmons' work it has been wrongly assumed that the sodium content of citrated blood might carry the risk of causing intraventricular haemorrhage when exchange transfusion is carried out. Table III shows that the added sodium load during a 200 ml/kg exchange transfusion with blood containing 168 mmol sodium per litre, is 2.8 mmol per kilogram (the load would be less than this if the sodium concentration of the blood withdrawn rose during the transfusion). Simmons et al considered that a single bolus injection of sodium bicarbonate containing less than 8 mmol/kg sodium could be considered safe. In exchange transfusion with citrated blood we thus have a situation where a sodium load that would be considered safe if given as a single acute injection is given slowly over a period of two hours. After a 90% exchange transfusion using blood with a sodium content of 168 mmol/l, the theoretical plasma concentration in the infant transfused would be 165 mmol/l. In practice the plasma sodium concentration in the infant does not change during exchange transfusion (Table III) presumably due to the fact that the slowness with which the sodium load is added allows equilibration effects to occur.[4,5]

During simple top-up transfusion with packed cells the sodium load to the infant is trivial and of no consequence.

TABLE III

SODIUM LOADING IN EXCHANGE TRANSFUSION

Plasma sodium in citrated blood (50 samples 24-72 hrs old)	168 mmol/l
Sodium (plasma) load per	
20 ml exchange (PCV 50%)	= 1.68 mmol
less (withdrawn)	= 1.40 mmol
	0.28 mmol
∴ Sodium load per kg at 200 ml/kg exchange	= 2.8 mmol
Theoretical plasma sodium at end of exchange transfusion	= 165 mmol/l

21 Exchange transfusions - Infants' Plasma Sodium (mmol/l)

Pre-exchange	Post-exchange
138 ± 6	139 ± 4

Neonatal hypocalcaemia induced by citrate is not a disorder with any significant long-term effects even when it causes convulsions.[2] In the short term it can usually be corrected by calcium gluconate. During exchange transfusion we give 1 ml of 10% calcium gluconate per 100 ml of blood exchanged, and in a series of 21 exchange transfusions found that the babies' pre-transfusion serum calcium concentrations had a mean value of 2.09 and a post-transfusion value of 2.23 mmol/l.

Citrated blood, stored for 24-48 hours, after which interval it is often used for neonatal transfusion carries less risk of infection than heparinised blood which has to be used fresh. The risk in exchange transfusion of infecting the infant with cytomegalovirus in particular seems to be considerable[9] (Table IV).

TABLE IV

CMV ISOLATION

Type of Case	No.	Virus Isolated	Frequency
Routine hospital admissions first year of life	935	28	3%
SCU follow up cases - no exchange transfusion	42	nil	nil
SCU follow up cases - exchange transfusion	51	15	29%

SCU = Special Care Unit (Newborn)

(After Tobin et al 1975)[9]

There has been a dramatic drop in the number of exchange transfusions in recent years (Fig. 1). The great majority of transfusions are now simple top-up transfusions in which citrate effects are of little significance.

Figure 1

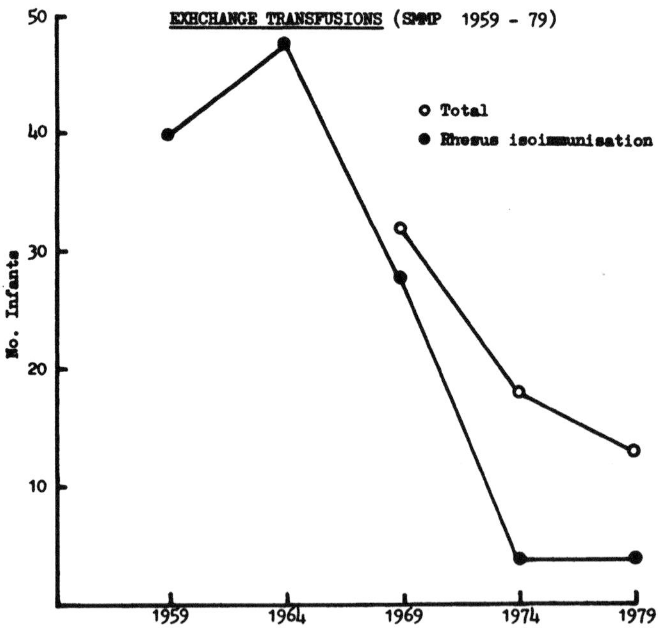

While anticoagulation with heparin in accepted therapeutic dosage is unlikely to cause bleeding in the presence of a normal platelet count, the same degree of heparinisation in the presence of thrombocytopenia carries a risk of induced bleeding. Thrombocytopenia is often present in the type of infant requiring exchange transfusion.

TABLE V

SMMP 1979

TRANSFUSIONS IN NEWBORN INFANTS

Total live-born infants		4906
Total infants given top-up transfusion		
single transfusions	46	
multiple transfusions	74	120
Total top-up transfusions given		259
Total infants exchange transfused (4 Rh: 4 infections: 2 ABO: 2 unexplained jaundice: 1 prematurity)		13
TOTAL EXCHANGE TRANSFUSIONS		20

Heparin causes a significant rise in free fatty acids in the newborn infant and these compete with bilirubin for albumin binding sites.[6] Thus, where exchange transfusion is being performed to reduce hyperbilirubinaemia, displacement of bound bilirubin from albumin by free fatty acids could have an adverse effect.

Because heparinised blood has to be used shortly after it is obtained, this type of preservation involves more wastage of blood than does citration and also, because it has to be used fresh, involves special donor bleeding arrangements.

No matter what type of blood is used, transfusion of the infant, particularly exchange transfusion, is a procedure requiring considerable technical skill which should only be carried out by those who maintain a continuing experience in the procedure and in centres where proper facilities exist in the form of a paediatric medical and nursing team working closely together and collaborating with an established blood transfusion service.

BLOOD TRANSFUSION IN PAEDIATRIC PRACTICE

Blood transfusion can be a single sporadic event or a procedure which has to be repeated over and over again for months or years. It can be used to augment a patient's existing blood supply or in exchange transfusion to replace it; it can be used to make good qualitative deficiencies. Among the specialities of surgery, medicine, obstetrics and paediatrics blood transfusion is one of the most widely used and valuable therapeutic procedures.

TABLE VI

BLEEDING DISORDERS IN CHILDHOOD
FOR WHICH BLOOD TRANSFUSION MAY BE REQUIRED

Trauma	D I C
Repeated blood sampling	Idiopathic thrombocytopenic purpura
Post-operative	Glanzmann's disease
Oesophageal varices	Thrombotic thrombocytopenia
Oesophageal hiatus hernia	Thrombocytopathia
Peptic ulceration	Bernard Soulier syndrome
Aspirin	May-Hegglin anomaly
Meckel's diverticulum	Hermansky Pudlak syndrome
Anaphylactic purpura	Wiskott-Aldrich disease
Haemorrhagic disease of the newborn	Haemophilia (VIII)
Feto-maternal haemorrhage	Christmas disease (IX)
Twin-twin transfusion	Congenital afibrinogenaemia (I)
Haemorrhagic telangiectasia	Congenital dysfibrinogenaemia (I)

Factor V (proaccelerin) deficiency
Factor VII (proconvertin) deficiency
Factor X (Stuart Prower) deficiency
Factor XI (PTA) deficiency
Factor XIII (fibrin stabilising) deficiency
Von Willebrand's disease
Heparin therapy

A discussion of blood transfusion in paediatrics inevitably leads us to a consideration of the conditions in which blood transfusions are recognised to have a therapeutic role. In practical terms blood, as such, is necessary in three main types of disorder:

1. acute blood loss with exsanguination;
2. haemolysis with rapid blood destruction;
3. anaemia,

whether due to inadequate red cell haemoglobinisation, as in iron deficiency anaemia, chronic blood loss, reduced red cell survival as in prematurity, or inherent defects in red cells as in spherocytosis or G-6-PD deficiency.

Table VI lists some of the childhood disorders in which blood loss from haemorrhage may occur either acutely or chronically and necessitate use of blood transfusion as a therapeutic measure - in some disorders probably once only, in others on an oft repeated basis. Three broad groups are evidenced. Firstly, rupture of blood vessels may result either from obvious physical injury or from disease, particularly disease of the alimentary tract. Secondly, platelet

TABLE VII

ACUTE HAEMOLYTIC DISORDERS IN CHILDHOOD
FOR WHICH BLOOD TRANSFUSION MAY BE REQUIRED

Spherocytosis	Sickle cell disease
Elliptocytosis	Thalassaemia
Infantile pyknocytosis	
Stomatocytosis	Auto-immune haemolytic disease
Congenital dyserythropoietic anaemia	Neonatal haemolysis due to infection
Heinz body anaemia of newborn	Rh incompatibility
G-6-PD deficiency	Haemolytic ureamic syndrome
6-PGD deficiency	Malaria (falciparum)
Glutathione reductase deficiency	Severe burns
Glutathione peroxidase deficiency	Radiation
Glutathione synthesis deficiency	Intracardiac prostheses
Pyruvate kinase, etc. deficiency	

deficiencies or defects, and thirdly, coagulation defects may lead to spontaneous bleeding or intractable bleeding from insignificant trauma.

Table VII indicates a number of haemolytic disorders in infancy and childhood where blood transfusion may be necessary. In group terms these could be described as disorders of red cell structure (eg, spherocytosis), disorders of red cell chemistry, particularly enzymatic deficiencies (eg, G-6-PD deficiency), haemoglobinopathies (eg, thalassaemia) and a variety of circumstances in which normal red cells are destroyed by external agencies, (eg, burns).

TABLE VIII

CHILDHOOD ANAEMIAS
FOR WHICH BLOOD TRANSFUSION MAY BE REQUIRED

Iron deficiency	Haemolytic anaemias
Disturbance of folate metabolism	Acquired
Prematurity	Congenital
Infection	Haemoglobinopathies
Malabsorption	
Haemolysis	Anaemia of prematurity
Nutritional deficiency	Anaemia of chronic infection
Anticonvulsants	Anaemia of collagen disease
Inborn errors	Anaemia of renal disease
Increased loss	Anaemia of liver disease
	Anaemia of endocrine disease
Vitamin B12 deficiency	Anaemia of malignant disease
Impaired absorption	
Nutritional	Anaemia secondary to thrombocytopenia or platelet defect
Aplastic anaemia	Congenital
Acquired	Acquired
Congenital	

(After Willoughby 1977)[10]

Anaemia is an extremely common disorder in childhood. It may result from deficiency of the elements, such as iron, necessary for the normal formation of blood, from hereditary or acquired inability to form blood cells (eg, Fanconi's anaemia), from sub-acute or chronic haemolysis (eg, leukemia) or from a number of states which depress the formation of blood red cells (eg, infection) or increase the rate of destruction (eg, prematurity). These broad categories are indicated in Table VIII. Lists of this sort indicate the enormous range of disorders for which blood transfusion may be a necessary and at times the only effective type of therapy available.

BLOOD TRANSFUSION AND THE NEWBORN INFANT

Neonatology is one of the most rapidly expanding branches of medicine and one which exemplifies well the increasing significance of the blood transfusion service in paediatric practice. The newborn infant is peculiarly prone to bleed in view of the traumatic circumstances of birth, the fragility of neonatal vessels, the deficiencies in clotting mechanisms and the raised venous pressure which is often present. It has been estimated[3] that bleeding is a primary cause of 5% of neonatal deaths and a secondary cause in a further 4%. The antigenic relationship which can exist between fetus and mother can result in haemolytic disease which may also arise from the fact that the fetus is so often the unwitting repository of drugs that have been consumed by his mother.

In neonatal practice, the restitution of blood lost by simple transfusion may be necessary as a result of fetal bleeding into the maternal circulation, spontaneous transfusion from one twin to another, incision of a placental or a cord vessel during Caesarean section, bleeding from the stump of the umbilical cord, repeated blood sampling especially in the low birthweight infant, haemorrhagic disease of the newborn associated with low prothrombin levels, internal bleeding from the cranium (eg, subdural, subarachnoid, intraventricular), or from abdominal organs (eg, subcapsular in the liver). Asphyxia, so common in the neonatal period, will increase the liability to bleeding by raising venous pressure. Disseminated intravascular coagulation is a hypercoagulable state peculiarly liable to occur in the newborn infant as a result of hypoxia, acidosis, hypothermia, infection, Rh incompatibility, birth injury and polycythaemia, and to be followed by a hypercoagulable state and bleeding due to consumption of platelets and clotting factors. Thrombocytopenia may also occur as an isolated deficiency. Deficiency of Factors VII, IX and X impairs clotting. Immaturity in association with low birth results in even greater fragility of the blood vessels.

Exchange transfusion is performed more frequently in the newborn infant than at any other age period - in cases of haemolytic disease of the newborn resulting from Rh incompatibility, hyperbilirubinaemia, overwhelming infections not responding adequately to antibiotic or chemotherapeutic agents and in prematurity with a view to improving respiratory exchange.

The current pattern of transfusion practice in neonatalogy is shown in Table V and Figure 2.

Figure 2

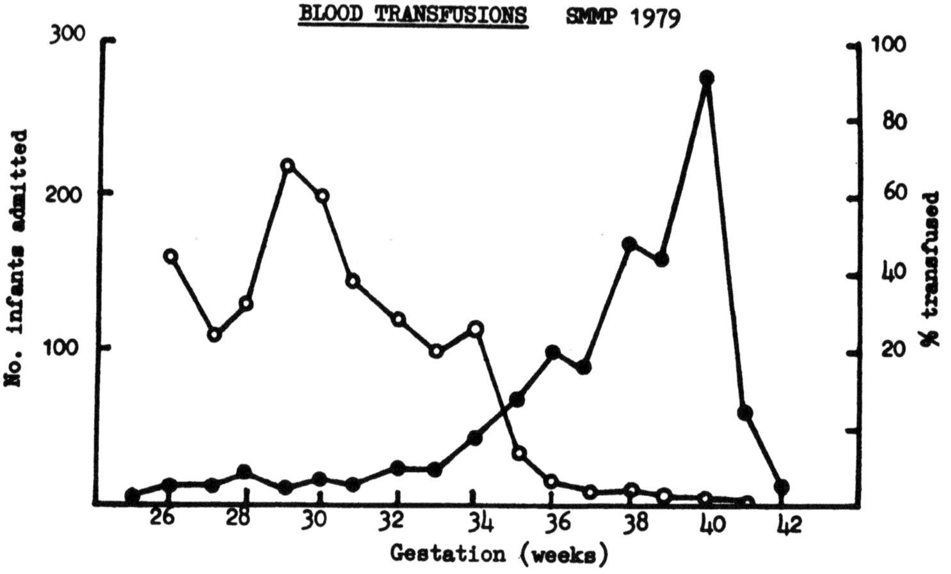

Thus, approximately 1 in 40 newborn infants received blood transfusions, two-thirds of these receiving multiple transfusions. The ratio of simple top-up transfusion to exchange transfusion was 13 to 1. The relationship of transfusion to gestation is shown in Figure 2 which indicates that a high proportion of infants of short gestation (low birthweight) require transfusion (eg, 90% of infants of 28-30 weeks gestation) while only a small proportion of infants of full gestation do so. In the short gestation (low birthweight) infants, the main aetiological factor is the blood sampling necessary for the biochemical monitoring of such infants.

Table IX shows that approximately 1 in 100 infants was given blood products for coagulation defects. Figure 3 shows the extent to which coagulation defects requiring blood products occur in short gestation (low birthweight) infants, with 6 out of 10 infants of gestational age 24-27 weeks requiring blood products.

Figure 3

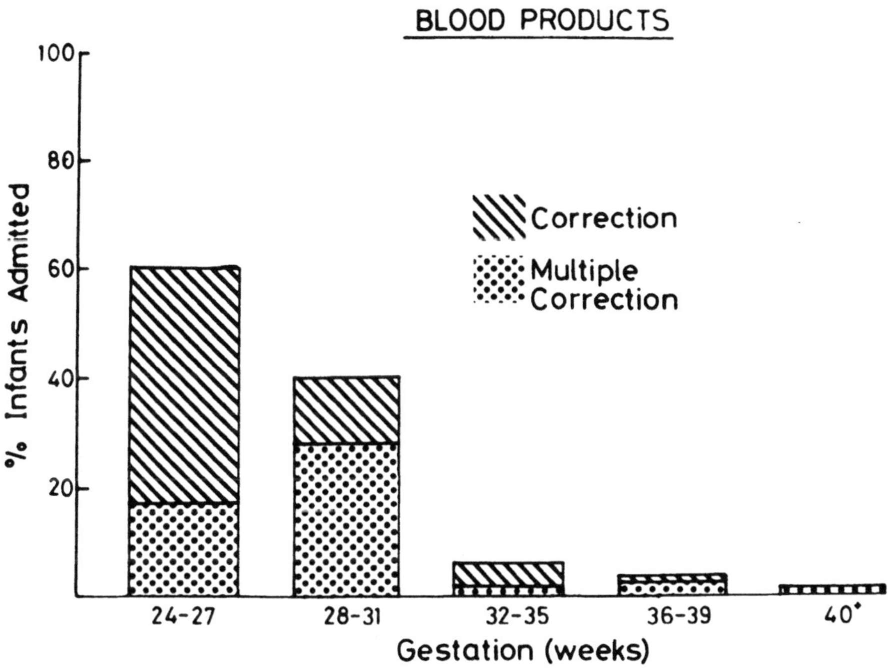

TABLE IX

SMMP 1979

BLOOD PRODUCTS USED - NEWBORN INFANTS

Total liveborn infants		4906
Total no. infants receiving blood products		
single administrations	23	
multiple administrations	27	50
Infants receiving:-		
Fresh frozen plasma		40
Cryoprecipitate		17
Platelets		11
Factor concentrate		11

BLOOD TRANSFUSION RISKS

Few, if any, effective forms of therapy are without risks and complications and blood transfusion is no exception. In paediatrics, unlike adult medicine, we are dealing with patients who exhibit a very wide range of blood volume, and the possibility of volume overload, particularly in the newborn infant, requires careful calculation of transfusion volumes. Haemolytic transfusion reactions can occur at any age but the less well developed immunological status of the newborn infant makes them less likely at this time. With effective blood grouping and cross matching, transfusion with blood mismatched from an ABO point of view is unlikely to occur but even if it does there may be little in the way of transfusion reactions. Rarely donor cells of other blood groups (eg, Lewis) may be slowly lysed by lytic antibodies in the recipient. Haemolysis of transfused red cells may also occur when they have been damaged by osmosis (as the result of some defect in the preserving fluid), by overheating, by freezing or by injection under pressure. An immediate febrile reaction is often associated with destruction of red cells in the patient's reticulo-endothelial system, and there may be a later fall in haemoglobin level. The result of serious haemolysis will be haemoglobinaemia with a possibility of renal failure and the development of disseminated intravascular coagulation. Delayed haemolytic transfusion reactions occur usually about a week after transfusion and may include jaundice, haemoglobinaemia or haemoglobinuria.

HLA antigens on leucocytes, platelets and in plasma, and apparently other antigens outside the HLA system, may also produce transfusion reactions. These may take the form of an immediate febrile reaction shortly after the commencement of the transfusion or post-transfusion thrombocytopenia usually one week after transfusion. Anaphylactoid reactions may occur rarely as a result of antigen/antibody reactions between immunoglobulins.

The introduction of infection is a possible risk of transfusion. The most serious is likely to be viral infection leading to viral hepatitis although the introduction of screening tests for Australia antigen has resulted in a significant decline in the risk of transmitting hepatitis B. The virus of hepatitis A,and non-A non-B hepatitis, can be transmitted by transfusion as can viruses of infectious mononucleosis, cytomegalovirus (Table IV), herpes simplex virus and Epstein-Barr virus. Bacterial contamination of transfused blood, reactions due to pyrogens, and the transmission of protozoa (eg, malaria) are other possible transfusion hazards.

Chemical toxicities may also occur. Citrate toxicity with a lowering of the level of ionised calcium has already been referred to as a hazard in exchange transfusion. Phosphorous loading in CPD blood may aggravate this. ACD blood being acidic may aggravate the base deficit which is often present in children, particularly infants. Haemolysis in the transfused blood may result in potassium toxicity. Hypoglycaemia may occur as a result of insulin response engendered by the high glucose load in the transfused blood. Apart from the transfused fluid itself, the possibility that plasticisers from the containers and tubing may have a toxic effect has been raised. In particular, di-2-ethyl hexyl phthalate (DEHP) has been incriminated as a possible cause of necrotising enterocolitis. Thrombophlebitis may develop as a local reaction in the vein used for transfusion.

Transfusion with blood in the ice-cold state may cause ventricular arrhythmias.

A particular problem with children who require repeated transfusions is that of transfusion haemosiderosis. One litre of blood contains approximately 500 mg of iron which is several hundred times the normal daily excretion of urine. Fortunately, continuous infusion of desferrioxamine over several hours, several times a week or by frequent subcutaneous injection holds out promise that iron excretion can be sufficiently increased to balance the input in patients such as those suffering from thalassaemia who require repeated blood transfusions over long periods of time.

The list of adverse reactions to blood transfusion is long. Some of the complications can be serious. Despite this, in competent hands the incidence of adverse transfusion reactions in children is probably considerably less than the 5 per cent given for transfusions in general, and most of the reactions are relatively mild.

REFERENCES

1. Anderson, J.M., Bain, A.D., Brown, J.K., Cockburn, F., Forfar, J.O., Machin, G.A. and T.L. Turner: Hyaline membrane disease, alkaline buffer treatment and cerebral intraventricular haemorrhage. Lancet, 1:117, 1976.
2. Brown, J.K., Cockburn, F. and J.O. Forfar: Clinical and chemical correlate in convulsions in the newborn infant. Lancet, 1:135, 1972.
3. Chamberlain, R. et al: First Week of Life. British Births vol.1, Heinemann, London, 1960, p.241.
4. Corbet, A.J., Adam, J.M., Kenny, J.D. et al: Controlled trial of bicarbonate therapy in high risk premature newborn infants. J.Paed. 91:771, 1977.
5. Finberg, L.: The relationship of intravenous infusions and intracranial haemorrhage: a commentary. J.Paed. 91:777, 1977.
6. Milner, R.D.G.: Neonatal Metabolism and Endocrinology Studied by Exchange Transfusion in Clinics in Endocrinology and Metabolism. ed. J.O. Forfar, W.B. Saunders, London, Philadelphia, Toronto, 1976, p. 221.
7. Mollison, P.L.: Blood Transfusion in Clinical Medicine. Blackwell Scientific Publications, Oxford, London, Edinburgh, Melbourne, 1979.
8. Simmons, M.A., Adcock, E.W., Bard, H. and F.C. Battaglia: Hypernatremia and intracranial hemorrhage in neonates. New Engl.J.Med. 291:6, 1974.
9. Tobin, J.O'H., Macdonald, H. and M. Brayshay: Cytomegalovirus infection and exchange transfusion. Brit.med.J. 2:404, 1975.
10. Willoughby, M.L.N.: Paediatric Haematology. Churchill Livingstone, Edinburgh, London, New York, 1977.

----

2. PRACTICAL ASPECTS OF EXCHANGE TRANSFUSION

T.L. TURNER

In common with other paediatric departments in the United Kingdom we have been aware of a significant decrease in the incidence of infants with haemolytic disease of the newborn (HDN), and as a result of this fall and the use of alternative methods of treatment the need for exchange transfusions in infants with HDN has fallen dramatically. In the three year period 1968–70, 50 infants required exchange transfusions for HDN, 94 exchange transfusions being performed (Table I).

TABLE I

EXCHANGE TRANSFUSIONS

	H D N	Non H D N
1968 - 70	50 (94)	9 (11)
1977 - 80	12 (16)	16 (17)

The number of exchange transfusions for each individual varied from one to a maximum of five. These figures represent an incidence of exchange transfusion for HDN in Hull of 5 per 1,000 liveborn infants in that period. During the same period, 9 infants required exchange transfusion for non-HDN reasons, a total of 11 exchange transfusions being performed. Comparative figures for the three year period 1977–80 from the same maternity hospital whose total births did not significantly alter revealed an HDN exchange incidence of 1.2 per 1,000 live born infants (Table II). In the latter period 12 infants required exchange transfusion for HDN and 16 exchanges were performed. During the same period 16 infants had 17 exchange transfusions performed for non-HDN indications. It is evident from the fourfold reduction in the number of infants requiring exchange transfusion for HDN and the sixfold reduction in the frequency of exchange transfusion that the facility to gain expertise in the performance of exchange transfusion is likely to become more difficult and that in any individual centre the number of physicians with the required training to perform exchange transfusions will likewise diminish.

TABLE II

INCIDENCE OF EXCHANGE TRANSFUSION

FOR RHESUS DISEASE IN HULL

1968 - 70	- 5/1000
1977 - 80	- 1.2/1000

The majority of infants who require exchange transfusion for HDN will do so either because of anaemia or hyperbilirubinaemia or a combination of both. There will, however, be a smaller number more severely affected who will have haematological evidence of disseminated intravascular coagulation (DIC), and exchange transfusion will contribute a further dimension to their management.

Our indications for exchange transfusion in Hull have not changed significantly in the past 10 years and are similar to those used in other centres in the United Kingdom (Table III). A primary indication is the presence of

TABLE III

INDICATIONS FOR EXCHANGE TRANSFUSION

FOR RHESUS DISEASE IN HULL

1. Cord haemoglobin < 10 gm
2. Cord bilirubin > 60 mmol/l
3. Hyperbiliribinaemia

hydrops or a cord haemoglobin less than 10 g/dl. We anticipate such severely affected infants where there is a rising maternal antibody level or after information from amniocentesis. Infants are also likely to be severely affected when plasmapheresis has been necessary or the fetus has had an intrauterine transfusion. Our experience with the latter two clinical situations is limited. We anticipate all known HDN deliveries and have available on the delivery ward a partially packed unit of Group O Rhesus negative citrated blood. This blood is between 24 and 72 hours old. A further indication for exchange transfusion at an early stage is a cord serum bilirubin of greater than 60 mmol/l or a serum bilirubin which is rising rapidly (eg, at a rate of greater than 10 mmol/l/hr). We utilise a standard graph to aid our decision for exchange in hyperbilirubinaemia but additionally consider that the following clinical features should weight our exchange decision:

Severe perinatal asphyxia
Metabolic acidosis
Hypothermia
Birth weight of under 1500 g
Respiratory distress syndrome.

When exchange transfusion is indicated we utilise one of four techniques:

1. Early partial exchange (up to 20-60 ml/kg) for severe HDN using fresh (less than 72 hrs old) citrated blood via the umbilical vein.
2. Two volume exchange (160 ml/kg) with fresh citrated blood using the umbilical vein in well term infants.
3. Two volume exchange with fresh citrated blood via umbilical artery and vein in low birth weight infants.
   We also use this technique in compromised term infants.
4. Two volume exchange with fresh heparinised blood in infants with established coagulation defects.

We are aware of the disadvantages of citrated blood and in particular the calcium and magnesium binding of citrate and the risks of acid base imbalance. However, by using fresh citrated blood the risks are reduced and we have not experienced significant acid base disturbance in infants transfused using this type of blood. To control symptomatic hypocalcaemia we give 1 ml of 10% calcium gluconate by slow infusion after each 100 ml of exchange blood in second and subsequent exchanges, but not during the first exchange. It is unusual to provoke hypoglycaemia during exchange transfusion with citrated blood and hyperglycaemia usually occurs. However, we monitor the blood glucose following exchange transfusion with ACD blood because of the risk of late reactive hypoglycaemia. The principal advantage of citrated blood is that it can be stored for periods of longer than 24 hours if necessary, and that neither interferes significantly with the coagulation state of the infant unlike heparinised blood. We do, however, use fresh heparinised blood where there is an established coagulation abnormality in an attempt to correct disseminated intravascular coagulation and when using this form of anticoagulated blood we have seen hypoglycaemia develop during the exchange, and now take steps to monitor the blood glucose during the procedure (Table IV). In infants who do

TABLE IV

CITRATED BLOOD

Advantages	Disadvantages
Longer storage	Calcium binding by citrate
Less interference with coagulation	Hypoglycaemia post exchange
No hypoglycaemia during exchange	Acid-base balance

not have coagulation defects the use of heparinised blood may provoke a coagulation abnormality which will require to be reversed by the use of protamine sulphate. Most infants will metabolise heparin within 6-8 hours, although very sick infants may take significantly longer. In addition to requesting fresh citrated blood compatible with mother's blood we are usually provided with blood which is low in anti A and anti B antibodies.

Prior to exchange, we attempt to correct asphyxia, hypoglycaemia, acidosis and hypothermia, and the infant's temperature, respiratory and cardiac status is monitored during the procedure which is performed under a radiant heater or in an incubator. It is essential that blood for exchange is heated adequately throughout the whole procedure and we use a coil and warmer preset to provide blood at a temperature of 37°C. The infant's stomach is aspirated before the procedure and the infant is not fed during or for several hours after the exchange. Where an umbilical arterial catheter is to be used this is inserted first using a sterile procedure. Having cannulated the umbilical vein it is then our custom to measure the central venous pressure and to use this as a guide to the working deficit if indicated during the exchange. It is our policy that the aliquot of blood used for each exchange should not exceed 10% of the estimated blood volume of the infant and we usually begin with 10 ml aliquots, increasing as the exchange proceeds to 20 ml if the infant weighs more than 2000 g. The rate of exchange has little effect on the amount of bilirubin removed[4] and most exchanges can be completed within 1 - 1½ hours irrespetive of which technique is used. Where the infant is at term and robust we usually exchange using only the umbilical vein, and a single operator uses an uncomplicated 'push pull' technique. However, in infants of lower birth weight or infants who are unwell we frequently use both umbilical artery and vein. Exchange transfusion can be performed with two operators, one inserting blood slowly into the umbilical vein in 10-20 ml aliquots, whilst the other removes a similar quantity from the umbilical artery. A modification of the technique described by Ata and Holman[1] uses a syringe pump to infuse donor blood into the umbilical vein whilst removing the infant's blood at the same rate manually via the umbilical artery. A further modification has automated the procedure further and was described by Philpott and Banerjee[3] in which an impeller pump of the Holter variety pumps blood into the umbilical vein and simultaneously removes it from the artery. This technique has been used on numerous occasions without complications once initial technical problems were overcome utilising a rate of 400 ml/hr in larger infants, or at half this rate in smaller infants. Utilising the umbilical artery and vein has the advantage of placing less strain on the infant and on the operator whilst blood volume variations are minimised.

Following exchange transfusion it is usual to remove both the umbilical and venous catheters, but where it is anticipated that further exchange transfusions may be required it is our practice to leave the umbilical arterial catheter in position. We do not routinely use prophylactic antibiotics, but will do so if the umbilical vein has to be cannulated on a second occasion or if the arterial catheter is left in situ for more than 24 hours. Following exchange transfusion we monitor the blood glucose at frequent intervals using Dextrostix and it is our practice to estimate blood serum electrolytes within the next 12 hours. We have not seen any significant biochemical disturbance apart from occasional hypocalcaemia, and have not experienced intracranial haemorrhage related to hypernatraemia as a complication of exchange transfusion. Following exchange transfusion it is usual for the serum bilirubin to fall to 50% of earlier levels, but this level quickly rises over the next two to three hours. The infant's haemoglobin is usually altered by exchange transfusion, the haemoglobin usually rising to 3-4 g/dl, particularly if partially packed blood has been used. Thrombocytopenia is common following exchange transfusion, but is of very short duration (usually less than 12 hrs) and seldom constitutes a clinical problem. Other important biochemical features are associated with the use of adult haemoglobin. These aspects are covered elsewhere in these proceedings.

In common with Chessels and Wigglesworth[2] we have also seen disseminated intravascular coagulation occur in rhesus immunised infants all of whom have had clinical haemorrhagic symptoms before exchange transfusion including the presence of petechiae, marked bruising and difficulty in controlling bleeding from injection sites. All of these infants were treated with exchange transfusion, using either heparinised or ACD blood. In most instances we see a rise in the plasma fibrinogen concentration and the platelet count following exchange transfusion, whilst the fibrin degradation product (FDP) usually falls. However, the effectiveness of exchange transfusion is short lived and may require to be repeated for continuing DIC. We have found it particularly difficult in evaluating other coagulation parameters when heparin has been used, and at the moment our preference is for fresh citrated blood.

Whilst the need for exchange transfusion in newborn infants with HDN has diminished, the expertise available to perform these procedures safely has also diminished and lends weight to the suggestion that rhesus immunised pregnancies should be managed on a centralised basis where possible. In our practice, where infants are stabilised before exchange transfusion takes place, citrated blood of less than 72 hours old has caused few difficulties and is still our blood of choice for routine exchange. The management of DIC in severely affected rhesus infants still poses a very significant management problem, part of which can at least be improved by the use of exchange transfusion.

REFERENCES

1. Ata, M. and C.A. Holman: Simultaneous umbilical arteriovenous exchange transfusion. Brit.med.J. 2:743, 1966.
2. Chessells, J.M. and J.S. Wigglesworth: Haemostatic failure in babies with Rhesus isoimmunisation. Arch.Dis.Childh. 46:37, 1971.
3. Philpott, M.G. and A. Benerjee: Automated method for exchange transfusion. Arch.Dis.Childh. 47:815, 1972.
4. Sproul, A. and L. Smith: Bilirubin equilibration during exchange transfusion in haemolytic disease of the newborn. J.Paed. 65:12, 1974.

3. INDICATIONS FOR EXCHANGE TRANSFUSION AND CHOICE OF TREATMENT FOR HAEMOLYTIC DISEASE OF THE NEWBORN

N.R.C. ROBERTON

Before discussing the contentious subject of the indications for exchange transfusion for jaundice in a patient with haemolytic disease of the newborn (HDN), I will consider the indications in very ill infants who are born anaemic, hydropic or prehydropic, following the administration of an intrauterine transfusion.

1. Hydrops Fetalis

All infants born hydropic should be treated, since the outcome for such infants is now very much better.[12] The delivery of a hydropic infant requires the full facilities of the neonatal intensive care unit, and early treatment must be based on the fact that the infant will have three major physiological problems:

a) respiratory failure due to pulmonary oedema, ascites and pleural effusions, and often hyaline membrane disease due to the coexistent prematurity.
b) Plasma volume depletion and generalised anasarca with pleural, peritoneal and occasionally pericardial effusions.
c) profound anaemia comprising oxygen transport to the tissues, and impairing clinical assessment of hypoxaemia.

Early management is therefore based on:-

a) assisted ventilation from birth in all infants followed immediately by the insertion of umbilical, arterial and venous catheters to allow for control of blood pressure, central venous pressure and blood gases, with correction of these if abnormal.
b) Drainage of effusions - done with great care since panic insertion of trocars into any body cavity can damage the viscera therein. This is particularly true with the hepatosplenomegaly of severe rhesus HDN.

c) Exchange transfusion initially to raise the haematocrit. A single volume exchange transfusion is usually adequate.

All this can be done within the first hour.

2. Anaemia

Infants with a cord haemoglobin of < 10G% should have an exchange transfusion within the first two hours of life; the further below 10G% the sooner, within those two hours, the exchange should be started. Infants with haemoglobins of < 6G% constitute a major neonatal emergency even if they are not hydropic.

With cord haemoglobin levels between 10G% and 12G% the infant will almost certainly need an exchange transfusion, or at least a top up transfusion. Many workers therefore feel that such infants should so be exchanged within the first few hours of life. Above 12G% of haemoglobin in cord blood the decision to exchange is based more on the bilirubin values and their rate of rise.

3. Infants post intrauterine transfusion

There is nothing special about the management of such patients. Points to note however are:

a) The cord results may be confusing with a large proportion of rhesus negative donor cells, and a comparatively large component of conjugated bilirubin.

b) If the intrauterine transfusion has not been absorbed, it needs to be aspirated taking the same proportions as when aspirating ascites of a hydropic infant.

c) The infant is often premature and must be scrutinised for the illnesses of prematurity - particularly hyaline membrane disease which has an increased incidence in infants with severe HDN.

4. Jaundice

In the mid 1950s when the technique for exchange transfusion for rhesus HDN became established[15] the general recommendation was that an exchange transfusion should be carried out to prevent the plasma unconjugated bilirubin level exceeding 20 mgm%. This data was based primarily on studies in babies weighing > 2.50 kg, and large retrospective studies on such infants show that kernicterus was unknown in infants with unconjugated bilirubin levels less than this, and indeed it was rarely seen with unconjugated bilirubin levels of 20-25 mgm%.[14]

However, in the last twenty-five years it has become clear that the plasma unconjugated bilirubin at which kernicterus may develop is much more variable. At one end of the spectrum, plasma unconjugated bilirubin may rise to 25 mgm% in asymptomatic mature infants without any signs subsequently of kernicterus or brain damage.[2] At the other end, kernicterus has been reported at postmortem in low birthweight short gestation infants dying from severe hyaline membrane disease, sepsis or intraventricular haemorrhage in whom there has been no clinical evidence in life of kernicterus, and in whom the plasma unconjugated bilirubin did not exceed 10 mgm%.[6,8] Furthermore, in follow up studies of surviving low birthweight infants, jaundice is one of the factors correlating with neurological sequelae in survivors[13] and the famous studies of Boggs' group[3,11] also suggested that jaundiced low birthweight survivors had more subtle neurological abnormalities in the first year of life than the non jaundiced.

Crucial in the evaluation of this data is an understanding of the pathochemistry of kernicterus.[4,5]

At pH of 7.40 unconjugated bilirubin is highly insoluble both in fat and water (water solubility 5 ng/100 ml), and the majority of unconjugated bilirubin in plasma is firmly bound to one high affinity site on albumin molecules. Only minute nanomole quantities of bilirubin are dissolved and free in the plasma. This bilirubin in solution is in equilibrium between the free bilirubin anion and the free bilirubin acid, the ratio being 10^6:1 at pH 7.40. It is the free bilirubin acid which is neurotoxic, and it probably exerts its effects by binding to membrane phospholipids including those of mitochondria, thereby poisoning their metabolic activities.

There is as yet no satisfactory method of measuring the amount of free bilirubin in plasma and particularly the amount of bilirubin acid, although methods of measuring the converse of free bilirubin, that is the reverse albumin binding capacity are satisfactory but as yet difficult to reproduce in different laboratories, and they have had little impact on clinical practice.[7] Nevertheless, based on the known binding constant of bilirubin for albumin, and the average concentration of albumin and bilirubin in infants with HDN who require exchange transfusion, it is possible to calculate that approximately 50 nmol of free bilirubin (primarily as the anion) will be present in the plasma of infants with unconjugated bilirubin levels in the 20 mgm% range, provided that no other chemical is present which might displace unconjugated bilirubin from its albumin binding site. The very small amount of bilirubin acid present in

50 nmol of free bilirubin at pH 7.50 does not cause kernicterus, but lowering the plasma pH increases the proportion of bilirubin acid which is present; at pH 7.05, sufficient free bilirubin acid is present to cause kernicterus when the total free bilirubin is only 10 nmol/L.

Based on clinical studies, various factors are known to increase the risk of kernicterus:-

Hyperalbuminaemia
Acidaemia
Hypoxia
Prematurity
Rapidly rising bilirubin
Hypoglycaemia
Sepsis
Drugs.

In general these work through either or both of two mechanisms:

1) They compete for bilirubin binding sites on albumin directly - as with drugs, or they increase plasma levels of free fatty acids, which are one of the major competitors for the bilirubin binding site.
2) They cause acidaemia which not only increases the amount of neurotoxic free bilirubin acid present, but also preferentially increases the binding of bilirubin (as the acid) to tissues rather than as the ionic form to albumin.

Clearly therefore, sick low birthweight premature infants have an increased risk of developing kernicterus. However, I am very unhappy about carrying out exchange transfusions at the very low levels of bilirubin recommended by some authors. For one thing, kernicterus found at postmortem when the plasma bilirubin level has never exceeded 10 mgm% must be an agonal event. All the factors which tend to increase free bilirubin acid will be at their most intense during the hour or so before death, and particularly during the 10-20 minutes of unsuccessful cardiopulmonary resuscitation which often intervenes between the infant's final clinical deterioration and certification of death. In support of this view is the the fact that the clinical sequelae of kernicterus such as athetoid cerebral palsy have not been described in surviving low birthweight infants whose bilirubin levels rose to equivalent levels.

Finally, the data relating minor neurological sequelae to neonatal jaundice is at best unconvincing because none of the studies adequately address themselves to the problem, that whatever it was that caused the increase in jaundice was also responsible for the subsequent mild neurological sequelae.

Putting all this data together, I do believe that it is reasonable to carry out exchange transfusions in premature infants at lower levels, and would recommend those in Table I which are based on the data of Pearlman et al[9].

TABLE I

PLASMA UNCONJUGATED BILIRUBIN AT WHICH TO CARRY OUT EXCHANGE TRANSFUSION IN INFANTS WITH RHESUS INCOMPATIBILITY

Birth weight (g)	Plasma bilirubin
< 1250	13 mgm %*
1250 - 1499	15 mgm %*
1500 - 1999	17 mgm %*
2000 - 2499	18 mgm %*
> 2500	20 mgm %*

*exchange should be carried out at levels 2-3 mgm less than this if the infant is seriously ill with acidaemia, hypoxia, septicaemia etc

The aim should always be to do the exchange transfusion before the unconjugated bilirubin values reach the levels shown in the Table, and serial 2 - 4 hourly measurements may be necessary. If the unconjugated bilirubin is rising at more than 0.5 - 1.0 mgm/hr then plans should be made in advance on the basis of the rate of rise to carry out the exchange transfusion before the danger level is reached.

CHOICE OF THERAPY IN HDN

The management of infants with HDN may require the full panoply of the techniques of neonatal intensive care, particularly if the infant is hydropic or premature. In this review, however, I will only cover the techniques used for the management of the hyperbilirubinaemia.

1. Exchange Transfusion

The techniques of exchange transfusion have been discussed elsewhere in these Proceedings and I will therefore only deal with which type of blood should be used.

Donor blood used In anticipation of delivery of the infant O Rhesus negative blood cross matched against the mother should always be available. If this is used, subsequent exchange should also be with O Rhesus negative blood irrespective of the infant's group. Some authorities recommend using O Rhesus negative blood in all situations, whereas others prefer to use ABO compatible blood if time allows this to be prepared after delivery and grouping of the infant.

If group O blood is used, some recommend using blood with a low titre of anti A and anti B, others resuspend the donor red cells in group AB plasma, while others say there is little point in carrying out either of these procedures. I know of no trial comparing these different recommendations, and there is much to be said for using the simplest technique of using ABO compatible blood if possible, and having O Rhesus negative always available for emergencies.

These is no place for the addition of A or B substances to the donor plasma, indeed if these are animal derivatives they have the potential for sensitising the infant to foreign protein.

Packed cells Since adult human blood has a lower haemocrit than that of normal newborn infants, and it is further diluted by the addition of the ACD or CPD, I believe that in most cases the donor blood should be partially packed before use.

Albumin Although giving albumin to the infant before the exchange transfusion does increase the amount of unconjugated bilirubin removed[16] there is no adequately controlled trial to show either that this practice reduces the risk of kernicterus, or reduces the number of exchange transfusions required. For this reason, and in view of the potential hazards from albumin infusion (fluid overload, hepatitis, confusing laboratory results), I do not feel that its use is justified.

Blood preservative anticoagulant Of the three alternatives available, ACD, CPD and heparinised blood, it is clear that ACD blood is an inappropriate fluid to infuse into infants. CPD blood is the only preservative that should be used for banking blood for neonatal use. The arguments still rage, however, about whether heparinised blood is preferable to CPD blood, because of the potential adverse metabolic effects of the latter. CPD blood may cause high plasma levels of sodium and potassium, it gives a citrate load with a potential for hypocalcaemia, and there is the risk of rebound hypoglycaemia following the exchange transfusion. Heparinised blood carries the small risk of heparinising the infant, and the heparin will increase plasma free fatty acid levels which will displace bilirubin from albumin. Opponents of heparinised blood claim enormous logistic problems in obtaining the blood fresh for the delivery of the infant or the next exchange transfusion, and complain about the wastage of this blood if it is not used.

The important question is however, whether the theoretical hazards of CPD blood actually materialise in clinical practice. For full term infants with Rhesus or ABO HDN who have minimal metabolic or cardiorespiratory disorders, are vigorous and active with normal blood gases, blood pressure, glucose and electrolyte values while breathing room air, CPD blood is perfectly safe.

Although there are no controlled trials to support either CPD blood or heparinised blood, I believe it is preferable to use heparinised blood in infants of $< 1.5 - 2.0$ kg who may be seriously ill, acidotic, septic, and in renal failure with or without coagulation disturbances. If CPD blood has to be used in such infants, most workers recommend that blood less than 24 hours old must be used because of the hazard of hyperkalaemia. The exchange must then be carefully paced to avoid the hypotension and collapse attendant on rapid exchange transfusion[1], the infant's pH should be measured once or twice during the exchange, and if it falls below 7.20 intravenous base should be given and the exchange halted for 15 - 30 minutes. The ECG should be monitored to look for hypocalcaemia which should be treated if it occurs. The infant's electrolytes should be checked post transfusion, and appropriate measures used to treat hyperkalaemia and hypernatraemia if they are present. Post transfusion hypoglycaemia should be sought by 2-hourly Dextrostix estimations for six to eight hours.

Although this level of monitoring and supervision will impose little stress on the type of neonatal intensive care unit in which such an exchange transfusion on small sick infants should be carried out, the fact remains that the CPD blood does pose an additional stress on the sick infant, in whom failure to attend to the minutiae of treatment can make the difference between neurologically intact survival on the one hand and death or handicap on the other.

2. Phototherapy

Phototherapy converts unconjugated bilirubin in the tissues by photo-isomerisation into bilirubin E which is water soluble, non-neurotoxic and can be excreted in the bile. In any infant in whom icterus develops due to Rhesus or ABO HDN, I believe that phototherapy should be given, since there is clear evidence that this reduces the number of exchange transfusions which have to be given subsequently (Table II).

Phototherapy is a powerful biological tool with many potentially serious side effects (Table III), not the least of which is unjustified mother-baby separation whilst the phototherapy is being given. I believe that in an otherwise well but jaundiced infant with HDN, the phototherapy should be given with the infant in a crib besides his mother. As soon as the bilirubin begins to fall the phototherapy can be discontinued.

3. Drugs

Although of considerable pharmacological interest, drugs which increase either bilirubin conjugation or gut transit time have no place in the management of HDN. They all take 24 - 48 hours to be effective, and their minimal potential benefit is grossly outweighed by their sedative or diarrhoea provoking side effects.

4. Fluid balance

An adequate fluid intake is essential, and in particular if phototherapy is being used, great care must be taken to make up for the increased fluid losses through gut and skin which are caused by this technique.

CONCLUSIONS

Immediate exchange transfusion should be carried out in all hydropic neonates and those with cord haemoglobin values < 10 G%. Subsequently exchange transfusion should be carried out to prevent the bilirubin reaching the values listed in Table I. CPD blood less than 48 hours old is suitable for most exchange transfusions, but in small sick infants heparinised blood is preferable. Jaundiced infants with Rhesus HDN should receive phototherapy and an adequate fluid intake plus any other supportive measures indicated. Drug treatment of such jaundice is unjustified.

Acknowledgement

I should like to thank my secretary, Miss Janita Whittingham, for her help in the preparation of this paper.

TABLE II

NUMBER OF EXCHANGE TRANSFUSIONS IN INFANTS RECEIVING PHOTOTHERAPY

No of Exchanges	Exchanges on Basis of Cord Blood		Exchanges for Hyperbilirubinaemia	
	P-THERAPY	NO P-THERAPY	P-THERAPY	NO P-THERAPY
0	14	38	32	32
1	31	40	9	20
2	-	-	3	13
3	-	-	-	7
4	-	-	1	5
5	-	-	-	1
	$p > 0.1$			$p < 0.01$

(Reid et al 1972)[10]

TABLE III

COMPLICATIONS OF PHOTOTHERAPY

1. OPTHALMIC	? RETINAL	
	CONJUNCTIVITIS	
2. FLUID LOSS	STOOLS	POOR WT GAIN
	TRANSEPIDERMAL	POLYCYTHAEMIA
3. THERMAL INSTABILITY	APNOEA	
	HYPOTHERMIA	
4. DERMATOLOGICAL	RASHES	
	BRONZING (CONJUGATED)	
5. INCREASED PERIPHERAL BLOOD FLOW		
6. ? PHOTOBIOLOGICAL EFFECTS		
7. MATERNAL ANXIETY/SEPARATION		

REFERENCES

1. Aranda, J.V. and A.Y. Sweet: Alterations in blood pressure during exchange transfusion. Arch.Dis.Childh. 52:545, 1977.

2. Bengtsson, B and J. Verneholt: A follow up study of hyperbilirubinaemia in healthy full term infants without isoimmunisation. Acta paediat.scand. 63:70, 1974.

3. Boggs, T.R., Hardy, J.B. and T.M. Frazier: Correlation of neonatal serum total bilirubin concentrations and developmental status at age eight months. J.Pediat. 71:553, 1967.

4. Brodersen, R.: Prevention of kernicterus, based on recent advances in bilirubin chemistry. Acta paediat.scand. 66:625, 1977.

5. Brodersen, R.: Bilirubin transport in the newborn infant reviewed with relation to kernicterus. J.Pediat. 96:349, 1980.

6. Gartner, L.M., Snyder, R.N., Chabon, R.S. and J. Berstein: Kernicterus: High incidence in premature infants with low serum bilirubin concentrations. Pediatrics 1970, 45:906, 1970.

7. Harper, R.G., Sia, C.G. and C.M.P. Kierney: Kernicterus 1980. Clinics in Perinatology 7:75, 1980.

8. Harris, R.C., Lucey, J.F. and J.R. Maclean: Kernicterus in premature infants associated with low concentrations of bilirubin in the plasma. Pediatrics 1958, 21:875, 1958.

9. Pearlman, L.A., Gartner, L.M., Leek, S., Morecki, R. and D.S. Horoupian: Absence of kernicterus in low birthweight infants from 1971 through 1976: Comparison with findings in 1966 and 1967. Pediatrics, 62:460, 1978.

10. Reid, M.C., McClure, G., Marks, E. and H.H. Elwood: Phototherapy in rhesus haemolytic disease. Lancet, 1972, p.879.

11. Scheidt, P.C., Mellits, P.C., Hardy, J.B., Drage, J.S. and I.R.Boggs: Toxicity to bilirubin in neonates: Infants' development during first year in relation to maximal neonatal bilirubin concentration. J.Pediatrics, 91:292, 1977.

12. Stewart, A.: Follow up of preterm infants in "Preterm Labour". Proc. 5th Study Group, roy.Coll.Obstetricians & Gynaecologists, ed: Anderson, A., Beard, R., Brudenell, J.M. and P.M. Dunn. Royal College of Obstetricians & Gynaecologists, London,1977, p.382.

13. Stewart, A.L. and E.O.R. Reynolds: Improved prognosis for infants of very low birthweight. Pediatrics, 54:724, 1974.

14. Walker, W., Ellis, M.I., Ellis, E., Curry, A., Savage, R.D. and R. Sawyer: A follow up study of survivors of rhesus haemolytic disease. Develop.Med.Child Neurol. 16:592, 1974.

15. Walker, W. and G.A. Neligan: Exchange transfusion in haemolytic disease of the newborn. Brit.med.J. i:681, 1955.

16. Waters, W.J. and E. Porter: Indications for exchange transfusion based upon the role of albumin in the treatment of hemolytic disease of the newborn. Pediatrics, 33:749, 1964.

4. PROGRESS IN EXCHANGE TRANSFUSION TECHNIQUES

M.M. KERR

Having studied the programme for the Symposium and having no wish to duplicate the advice given to other speakers, I decided that for the benefit of the younger members of the audience it would perhaps not be inappropriate to review briefly the whole intriguing subject of Rhesus incompatibility and its management. I will not take time to refer to the unravelling of the mysteries of aetiology, although that story is in itself a fascinating one, with inevitable arguments about who was really first to solve the problem. A study of the abundant literature does suggest that the credit should go to Levine and Stetson[9], who published their paper entitled "An unusual case of intra-group agglutination" in 1939. Although not strictly a comment on exchange transfusion as such, I quote the following passage from my own undergraduate paediatric textbook, under the heading "Familial Icterus Gravis".

> "The introduction of blood transfusion has superseded all other methods and has reduced the mortality in a remarkable way. Roughly 15 ml of blood should be given for each pound of the infant's weight, the transfusion being repeated if necessary every fourth or fifth day until the red cell count has returned to normal. Although the mother's blood is often used with eventual success, more satisfactory and lasting results may follow blood obtained from a donor outside the family, but recent investigations indicate that this will only be so provided the donor's blood does not contain the Rhesus factor, that is, is Rhesus negative, and a donor who is Rhesus negative should therefore be selected."[2]

No one should be alarmed! I am not suggesting this as a modern treatment for Rhesus incompatibility. I am quoting from "Diseases of Infancy and Childhood" by Wilfred Sheldon, 4th edition, published in 1943 and reprinted in 1945.[2] I was glad to find that, even as an undergraduate, I had written "NO" in red pencil against the suggestion that the mother's blood be used.

To paediatricians of my generation, 1943 does not seem all that long ago - but what enormous advances have been made since then in the management of Rhesus sensitised women and their babies - almost miraculously it seems - in the ability to prevent sensitisation even occurring.

To understand the advice given by Sheldon in 1943 we have to go back to 1932. In that year, Diamond and his co-workers in Boston published their classic Original Communication in the first volume of the Journal of Pediatrics.[5] This was entitled "Erythroblastosis fetalis and its association with universal edema of the fetus, icterus gravis neonatorum and anemia of the newborn". They quoted 173 references. One of the papers referred to, on universal oedema of the fetus, was by Ballantyne, a famous American obstetrician.[1] He had collected, or written up as we would now say, 70 such cases occurring between 1614 and the publication date of 1898.[1] This is the same Ballantyne who in 1901 published a paper entitled "A plea for a pro maternity hospital". In July of that same year, 1901, ONE bed was endowed in the Edinburgh Royal Maternity Hospital for the treatment of patients suffering from diseases of pregnancy.[8] Hitherto the patients had been admitted with great reluctance to the wards of the general hospitals. The fact that Louis Diamond was apparently unable to spell Edinburgh is of little consequence.

To return to Diamond. He and his co-workers told us that it was during the first two days of life that treatment was most effective. By treatment of course they meant the intravenous infusion of small amounts of blood. Their paper concluded with reports of 12 cases, 8 of whom survived.

I must now take a big jump to the year 1946. It was in that year that Wallerstein[14] devised a method of removing the Rhesus positive erythrocytes from the affected baby before they were destroyed in large numbers by the maternal antibody, and of replacing them with Rhesus negative cells. He described in this preliminary report simultaneous removal from the sagittal sinus and administration through a cannulated vein. Remarkably he also supported the alternative of removing 50 ml first, and then administering 50 ml. He described the procedure as dramatic and only submitted severely ill infants to the new regime. The next year - 1947 - produced two very important publications. Wallerstein[15] followed up his preliminary report and called the technique substitution transfusion. He indicated that for those who objected to withdrawing blood from the anterior fontanelle there were other sites available, including the radial artery. The method was to cannulate the artery and allow the blood to flow. My colleague Professor Charles Whitfield[16] tells me that he remembers vividly as an undergraduate in Belfast being detailed to catch in a galley pot the blood that was flowing from an incised radial artery. He commented that estimates of the volume so obtained were far from accurate.

To return to 1947. In that year Louis Diamond,[4] addressing the Royal Society of Medicine in London, also stressed that the removal of as much as possible of the affected infant's circulating blood shortly after birth seemed desirable. He too indicated that first attempts to do so were complicated by mechanical difficulties when using the anterior fontanelle and peripheral vessels. However, he then went on to describe the technique using a plastic catheter, of cannulating the umbilical vein, so facilitating what he called exsanguination transfusion. This would certainly seem to be the first description of what we now call a replacement or an exchange transfusion. It should not be forgotten, however, that another point was raised by Diamond in this communication. This of course was the question of planned early delivery when it seemed likely that the fetus was so severely affected that intrauterine death before term seemed inevitable. Remember that at this time the only guidance as to severity available to obstetricians was from the family history and the level of antibody titres.

Naturally the technique of performing exchange transfusions via catheterised umbilical veins gained rapid acceptance. In 1948, however, Mollison and Cutbush[11] are still cautious and write that the ability of this treatment to lower mortality and morbidity must still be considered unproven. Fortunately,a multi-centre trial was mounted by the Blood Transfusion Research Unit of the Medical Research Council. Although Belfast was involved, no Scottish centre was included. A preliminary report of the trial was published by Mollison and Walker in 1952.[12] I quote from the conclusions:

> Exchange transfusion was followed by a significantly higher survival rate than was simple transfusion, both treatments being carried out equally early after birth. The incidence of kernicterus after exchange transfusion was very low."

These observations were made on 477 cases of haemolytic disease, all born at 35 weeks gestation or later.

One might have hoped that rapid progress would have followed. However, in 1958 we read in a Lancet Editorial[6] that, despite what were called great strides, it was estimated that some 200 infants were still dying needlessly each year in England and Wales. It was emphasised that no new knowledge was required - only the application of that which now existed. The then Ministry of Health sent out a memorandum to all family doctors outlining the problem, particularly with regard to the importance of antenatal prediction of at-risk cases.

Also in 1958, Professor Forfar and his colleagues pointed out that the procedure of exchange was not entirely without risk, since sudden death could occur during the process.[7] Pleas were made for cases to be referred to large centres where expertise was high - some of us around that time were dealing with over 100 affected infants annually. This plea for referral was successful in some parts of the United Kingdom, but by no means in all. Even in the 1960s I was quite accustomed in my own department in Glasgow to have infants transferred from small hospitals after birth, with no warning at all, and certainly with no question of the vital prenatal discussion between obstetricians, paediatricians and the blood transfusion service. I am glad to say that this particular problem no longer exists in my area for a variety of reasons, not the least being the appointment of paediatricians with responsibilities in smaller obstetric units.

Other authors have given their personal views on the minutiae of techniques of transfusion and I must not be repetitive. But I should like to make it clear that in the West of Scotland, for practical reasons, it is not possible to obtain heparinised blood. Until a few years ago the anticoagulant used was acid-citrate dextrose (ACD). This has of course now been replaced by citrate phosphate dextrose (CPD). We find no problem, but are careful, particularly with preterm or very ill infants, to make frequent checks on the acid-base state, and we still use sodium bicarbonate as suggested by Barrie[2] in 1965.

It would be wrong to close this review without reference to mortality. Although selective early induction, amniocentesis, intrauterine transfusion and plasmapheresis have reduced perinatal mortality quite remarkably, for various reasons it will never be zero. McIlwaine and her colleagues,[10] surveying perinatal mortality in Scotland in 1977, found only 16 deaths attributable to Rhesus incompatibility out of a total of 1150 perinatal deaths relating to almost 63,000 births. Lastly, we would all wish to pay tribute to Sir Cyril Clarke, not only for his pioneering work in the use of anti-D, but for his continuing analyses of mortality in England and Wales.[3] His latest figures appeared in the British Medical Journal on 20 September 1980 and referred to the data for 1978: 93 infants were lost, 67 being stillborn and 26 born alive. The fact that in at least 28 of the cases there was no record of the at-risk mother being given anti-D means that in no way, even in 1980, may we become complacent about the problems of Rhesus incompatibility. Obviously there will still be cases requiring treatment for many years to come.

REFERENCES

1. Ballantyne, J.W.: Diseases of the Foetus. Edinburgh, 1898.
2. Barrie, H.: Acid base control during exchange transfusion. Lancet, ii:712, 1965.
3. Clarke, C. and A.G.W. Whitfield: Deaths from rhesus haemolytic disease in England and Wales in 1978: Accuracy of records and assessment of anti-D prophylaxis. Brit.med.J. ii:781, 1980.
4. Diamond, L.K.: Erythroblastosis foetalis or haemolytic disease of the newborn. Proc.roy.Soc.Med. 40:546, 1947.
5. Diamond, L.K., Blackfan, K.D. and J.M. Baty: Erythroblastosis fetalis and its association with universal edema of the fetus, icterus gravis neonatorum and anemia of the newborn. J.Pediat. 1:269, 1932.
6. Editorial: Haemolytic disease of the newborn. Lancet, ii:303, 1958.
7. Forfar, J.O., Keay, A.J., Elliot, E.D. and R.A. Cumming: Exchange transfusion in neonatal hyperbilirubinaemia. Lancet ii:1131, 1958.
8. Kerr, M.M.: A study of premature births in hospital. MD Thesis, University of Glasgow, 1956.
9. Levine, P., and R.E. Stetson: An unusual case of intra-group agglutination. J.Amer.med.Ass. 113:126,1939.
10. McIlwaine, G.M., Howat, R.C.L.,Dunn, F. and M.C. Macnaughton: Scotland 1977 Perinatal Mortality Survey. Univ.of Glasgow, 1979.
11. Mollison, P.L. and M. Cutbush: Exchange transfusion in haemolytic disease of the newborn. Lancet ii:522, 1948.
12. Mollison, P.L. and W. Walker: Controlled trials of the treatment of haemolytic disease of the newborn. Lancet, i:429, 1952.
13. Sheldon, W.: Diseases of Infancy and Childhood. J. & A. Churchill Ltd., London, 1945.
14. Wallerstein, H.: Treatment of severe erythroblastosis by simultaneous removal and replacement of the blood of the newborn infant. Science, 103:583, 1946.
15. Wallerstein, H.: Substitution transfusion: A new treatment for severe erythroblastosis fetalis. Ann.J.Dis.Childh. 73:19, 1947.
16. Whitfield, C.R.: Personal communication, 1980.

----

5. PRACTICAL EXPERIENCE IN NEONATAL EXCHANGE TRANSFUSION

C.A. HOLMAN

It was my good fortune to be concerned in blood transfusion in the early part of the second world war, then to be engaged in paediatrics and after that to become a pathologist at Lewisham. The unit there, under E.N. Allott, had started identifying Rh antibodies in 1941 and we developed a service for the whole of the London County Council hospitals. Up to 1947 we were in the unhappy situation of being able to diagnose haemolytic disease of the newborn and watch the natural course of the disease because, apart from simple transfusion, we were not able to treat it. Then in 1947 Diamond came to London to tell us about his combined treatment with induction of labour and exchange transfusion. Mollison at Hammersmith started to practise it, and Allott and I agreed to divide the London Area between the two units.

I shall now report on the results of our work and the changes we made in the practice of exchange transfusion.

Because Coombs did not develop his antihuman globulin test until 1945 there were a fair number of missed cases, chiefly with stillbirth or mild haemolytic disease. No special apparatus was available in those early days. Our catheters were cut from reels of polythene tubing intended to insulate telephone wires and were sterilised by boiling. The closed system we prepared connected the blood donor bottle, a heparinised saline bottle and a waste bottle via rubber and glass tubing and metal two-way taps to a syringe. Prophylactic penicillin was injected into the umbilical vein at the end of the exchange transfusion.

Despite the primitive nature of the procedure, the effects of a single exchange transfusion of 1 pint of Rh negative blood in an infant of 36 weeks maturity or weight of 2.5 kgs was remarkable. Survival increased by about 50%.

After a year interested British workers held a conference where the view was widely expressed that too many infants were being transfused and that transfusion was unnecessary unless the infant was anaemic. In the following period we transfused infants whose haemoglobin was below 14 gm/% and left those with higher levels. We were wrong! The kernicterus rate doubled and the extra cases were all babies having haemoglobin levels above 14 gm/%. In the earlier series no such babies had developed kernicterus. It may seem surprising, but in those days we did not know whether brain damage occurred before or after birth or was due to antibodies, bilirubin, or some other agent. These results, however, made it clear that kernicterus was preventable and was due to too high bilirubin levels.

When we reverted to transfusing all affected babies the kernicterus rate fell to its previous level. It was becoming clear that bilirubin levels above 20 mg/% carried a risk of kernicterus, and although various modifications of procedure were tried, it was not until 1952 that we realised we should leave the umbilical catheter in place and perform repeated exchanges as often as was necessary to keep the bilirubin level below 20 mg/%. Thereafter kernicterus was rarely seen. We did have a small epidemic when a penicillin resistant Staphylococcus entered the unit and felt obliged to change to streptomycin with penicillin prophylactically. But it became clear that this treatment carried a risk of deafness, and as erythromycin had become available we used it instead.

The other cases of kernicterus were largely due to late referral, with one exception in which an intradonor reaction occurred. An A_2 infant was exchanged with A_2 blood, then with A_1 blood, and then with O blood which was subsequently shown to have high titre immune anti-A antibodies. With a well organised scheme for the detection of antibodies during pregnancy and the referral of mothers to special centres we have not seen kernicterus for many years. The last case seen was due to an immune anti-A antibody with a super added infection and only occurred because of delay in recognising the jaundice and in referring the infant.

With the introduction of multiple exchange transfusion we also realised that we could reduce the risk to a severely affected fetus with congestive cardiac failure. Such infants have a raised venous pressure and an overloaded right heart and respiratory embarrassment. By replacing each sample of infant's blood with a lesser quantity of donor blood it is possible simultaneously to reduce the venous pressure, raise the haemoglobin and improve both the cardiac and respiratory states. Neonatal death from causes other that kernicterus was significantly reduced. This technique was exploited most successfully by David in Paris in his treatment of hydrops fetalis. A subsequent rise in neonatal deaths was the result of the much earlier induction of labour in our attempt to reduce the stillbirth rate.

Throughout the history of exchange transfusion there have been unexpected deaths in infants from cardiac arrest. There was no doubt in some cases that the catheter had entered the heart and in one case had passed into the left ventricle. In others the cause was not clear but we saw that cardiac arrest was more likely to occur with certain operators than with others and suspected that death was due to the mechanical effect of a jet of blood impinging on the myocardium. Ata and I then proposed the use of two catheters, one in the umbilical vein and the other in an umbilical artery. The donor blood flow in by gravity into the umbilical vein and the infant's blood flows out of the artery, the rate being adjusted to match the inflow. We had hoped that this would see the end of sudden deaths, but of course arterial catheterization produced problems of its own.

During the many years of exchange transfusion most of the infants who died did so from hydrops fetalis, respiratory disease, prematurity or a combination of these. A few were lost from infection and there were a number of rare causes. One infant who had a cardiac arrest actually died subsequently because of myocardial damage caused by cardiac massage. Another infant was lost because the catheter perforated the umbilical vein and caused a haemorrhage. The old polythene catheters had to be shaped before boiling: if a bevel was cut after boiling the point was like a spear. Congenital anomalies led to the normal proportion of neonatal problems and deaths.

The normal procedure for exchange transfusion was guided by bilirubin levels unless the clinical condition made earlier or later exchange advisable. We found it a great help to plot the haemoglobin and bilirubin levels on charts. Where information, eg, from antibody levels or amniocentesis, was available we might be prepared for severe disease. This was not always possible, as for instance in the case of immune anti-B haemolytic disease. We normally obtain suitable fresh blood of the infant's own ABO group in advance of induction, or in the case of ABO haemolytic disease suitable O cells and fresh frozen plasma. Originally the blood was collected in ACD but in recent years we have changed to CPD. We have never seen a need to use heparin. We like our blood to be 24 hours old and properly checked and we return it to the bank if not used at 72 hours. When we built our new special case baby unit we set up a small theatre with a laboratory next door so that progress could be monitored if necessary with blood levels.

Our success in recent years has been greatly improved by the arrival of neonatal paediatricians and by the development of the lecithin-sphingomyelin ratio which has stopped respiratory distress in deliberately induced babies.

6. EXCHANGE TRANSFUSION IN THE NETHERLANDS: A PERSONAL VIEW

P.C. DAS

It is four o'clock on a December morning and snow has been falling incessantly the whole night. In a hospital 50 km away an exchange transfusion is planned and fresh heparin blood of group O Rhesus negative is requested. A suitable donor has been called to the Donor Centre and blood was withdrawn by 4.45 a.m. As the blood was put on to an emergency taxi for transport information came that the baby had died. In this case it is unlikely that death could have been prevented and there is no doubt that the baby was acutely ill when first being considered for exchange transfusion. Time is a critical commodity here. The hospital concerned keeps a small stock of group O Rh negative blood which could have been made available within minutes from stock. A vital three-quarters of an hour could have been saved if stored Citrate Phosphate Dextrose (CPD) blood not more than 72 hours old had been acceptable.

My second case illustrates the human and scientific problems of such a situation. On an evening in November we were asked to supply fresh heparin blood for a Rhesus HDN baby of a mother with Rh antibodies anti CD in her serum at that point in time - and previously. Our own donor file is arranged positive or negative on the basis of presence or absence of the D antigen only. However, after a routine donation the Rh negative blood is further checked for the presence of C and other Rhesus antigens. A donor responded to our call at 10.0 p.m. but was not bled because of hypertension and low haemoglobin. A second suitable donor was found and blood withdrawn and sent directly to the Department of Paediatrics where it arrived at 11.30 p.m. By 2.0 a.m. the laboratory had reported cross matching difficulties with the donation which on investigation the next day it transpired were due to the presence of the C antigen. At about 3.0 a.m. the baby's serum bilirubin level was rising; the business of heparin blood was leading to nowhere! At that point the author persuaded the supervising paediatrician that there were 6 units of 48 hour old CPD blood in the bloodbank grouped for all Rhesus antigens and other tests.

These were likely to be suitable and would do for exchange transfusion as well if not better than heparin blood.

The advice was accepted and the exchange went through at 3.0 a.m. with good clinical results. The lesson to be learnt from this is that organising heparin blood is not only a problem of organisation but also involves the human element. The donor, being human, is subject to sickness and non-availability. In the situation described this was further complicated by the serology causing unusual delay. There is considerable risk in relying on a single unit of uncontrolled blood by a recipient known to have serum alloantibodies. Such a recipient is clearly defined as "dangerous". However, this extraordinary situation could easily have been avoided by accepting the CPD blood from the bank.

The third observation that I make in this saga is related to facets not generally appreciated by the expert medical world. A donor was called out at night and asked to report to the Donor Centre as soon as possible. To save a life he speeded up his driving and ice on the road landed him and his car on a nearby frozen canal; fortunately the accident was not serious.

A blood transfusion centre is not a magician, able to produce a suitable donor at the drop of a hat. The donors themselves are volunteers who wish to help society. But to subject them unnecessarily to physical and emotional risk is unacceptable. I must ask whether such heroic exploits are justified by their benefits when alternative treatment is quite clearly established and acceptable, clinically as well as scientifically.

These are the 1980s. We are on the verge of a new century. The formula for interferon has been agreed upon and in the not-too-distant future it may come to be more widely prescribed. One particular interferon is derived from human leucocytes harvested from buffy coat of donated blood, and so may be considered a blood product. This is one example of the scientific developments of the last two decades in blood transfusion practice that have played a significant role in patient care in almost all branches of clinical medicine. A simple concept of component policy in blood transfusion has been a major breakthrough; some of the potential has yet to be realised. It is simple - each therapeutic component is harvested, and when necessary given to the patients. Examples of cellular components include red cell concentrate, washed red cells and platelet concentrates; plasma components are fresh frozen plasma, cryoprecipitate and plasma fractionation products like Factor VIII, albumin and immunoglobulin.

Figure 1

INTERFERON AS A BLOOD COMPONENT

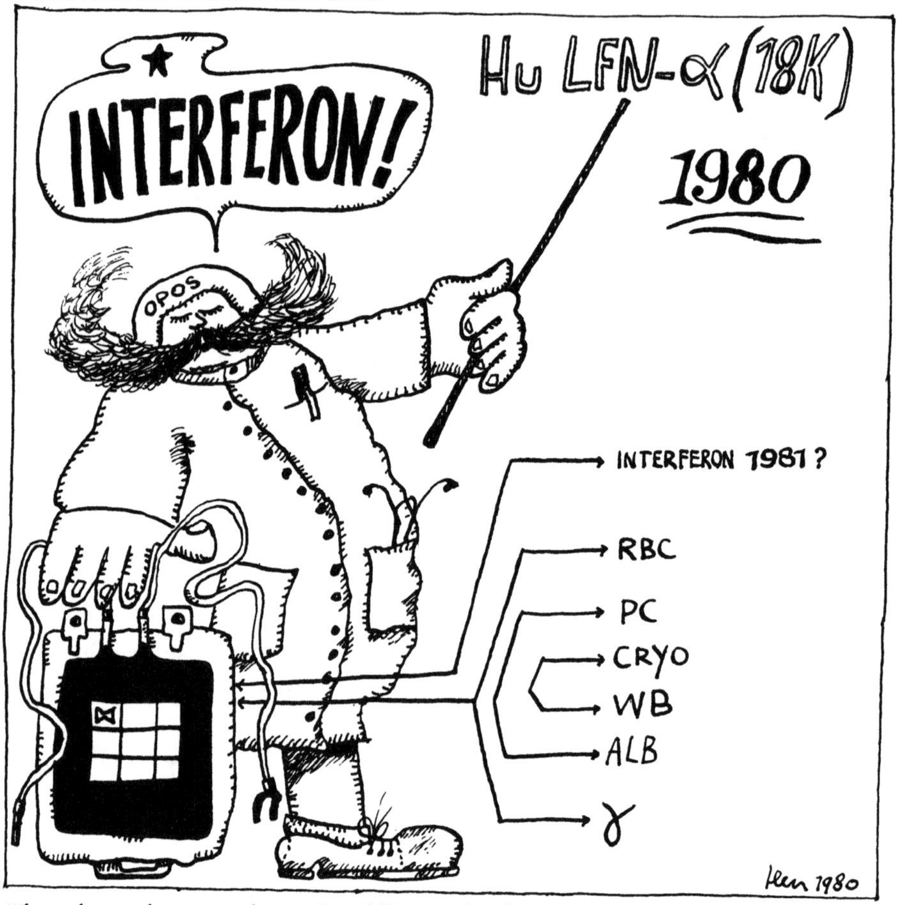

Why then the practice of adding animal substance to human blood for subsequent transfusion in the treatment of ABO incompatibility? Some paediatricians still demand that Witebsky-substance (or group A+B substance) be added to group O blood for use in exchange transfusion. The substance was first described by Witebsky in the 1940s while working in the Rockefeller Institute. He found that by treating the mother's blood with mucin from pigs and horses he could differentiate mothers whose babies were likely to be at risk. This in vitro test is based on the nature of antibody in the mother's serum, whether IgG or IgM. It was used as a laboratory test for a short time but by the mid-50s had been superseded by other biochemical methods.

In 1948, Queen Wilhemina reigned in the Netherlands; now her grand-daughter, Queen Beatrix, is Head of State. Man has landed on the moon. Genetic engineering is progressing for therapeutic products. Animals are happily being retired from the biological therapeutic field. In the blood transfusion service Acid Citrate Dextrose (ACD) as anticoagulant is being replaced by CPD, allowing better preservation of blood and its products, and plastic bags have permitted better component policy. Further, the introduction of cell separator machines in the blood banks has allowed the routine harvesting of enormous amounts of cells from a single donor - white cells, platelets and stem cells - unthinkable a decade ago. In this Region in the North of the Netherlands with its fourteen hospitals this modern therapeutic armoury allows us to provide a service to parallel modern patient care. (Table I)

TABLE I

THERAPEUTIC SUPPORT BY THE BLOODBANK GRONINGEN-DRENTHE FOR 3 YEARS

	1977	1978	1979
total donations	42917	45365	49257
cryoprecipitate	32169	26436	25606
platelets concentrate made	4803	5678	7690
platelets concentrate given	2294	3309	4765
loucocyte poor blood	4802	5805	6425
fresh frozen plasma made	2658	9792	11638
fresh frozen plasma given	2558	2619	3169
single donor plasma made	11330	12850	15804
single donor plasma given	3618	3529	3060
Cell Separator Unit			
thrombo pheresis	151	375	461
leucopheresis	52	111	88
plasma exchanges	209	326	238

Why then do we still receive requests for Witebsky-substance? Is this not a retrograde step? The answer may lie in the local system as it developed. Unlike the British and American systems where antenatal care is integrated with the blood transfusion service, in the Netherlands this is done by separate institutions which also do the cross matching. Another factor seems to be that most blood banks were formerly a part of the pharmacy service. Therefore the developments in the blood transfusion service did not filter through to the clinicians. Furthermore, in medical education and specialist training programmes there exists virtually no platform for the blood transfusion service to provide or pass on this specialist expertise and knowledge to colleagues. A simple example should suffice. For the routine collection of blood, a bacteriologically sterile and closed plastic bag system is used. Because of the lack of demand for heparinised blood bags in the Netherlands they are no longer available from the manufacturers. Thus, when heparin blood is requested, most blood banks have to open the closed system and remove the CPD anticoagulant and then inject a heparin solution into the bag. Despite aseptic handling there is no doubt that the sealed sterility is broken long before the withdrawal of blood. Some of these home made heparin bags may be stored for weeks and months. How many paediatricians are aware of this? Had this information been passed on and properly considered by those who seem to advocate mixing red cells with heparin plasma as a substitute, then they may have second thoughts. In addition to the risk of flocules formation[7] during the thawing of frozen plasma, the addition of plasma to red cells is a manoeuvre inviting potential pinhole injury to the bag.

One may ask what the Bloodbank Groningen-Drenthe has done recently to rectify the situation. Firstly, we have contacted and written to both haematologists and paediatricians all over the world. We have visited some of the paediatric units ourselves. Whilst I was not aware of the Handbook originating from the Harvard Medical School, or its publication date, I am well aware of the current exchange practice of the Children's Hospital Medical Center, Harvard Medical School, Boston as current in September 1980. I quote:[5]

> In instances where a neonate is suddenly transferred to our unit, and if an 'unpredicted situation' arises and exchange transfusion is necessary, we will convert CPD blood less than five days old to heparinized blood.
>
> Group specific blood is used for the infant in instances of Rh, K and Fy^a incompatibility, etc., provided there is no evidence of circulating anti-A or anti-B if the mother is of a different blood group than the baby.
>
> ABO compatibility: if the child is full term, we use group O

compatible blood that is negative for A and B hemolysins. If the child is premature, we use group O cells suspended in AB plasma. In those instances where the delivery is elective, and we are virtually sure that an exchange transfusion is to be performed, we will collect blood in heparin. (Donors are put on call.) Such infants included in this category are those who received intra uterine transfusions, infants delivered early because of past maternal history, or markedly rising amniocentesis findings during very late gestation.

Neonatal hyperbilirubinaemia without evidence of incompatibility: We use group and type specific; most often CPD blood is converted with heparin.

All blood for exchange transfusions must be less than five days old. We will go to seven days in an emergency."

Secondly, we have collected up-to-date literature and publications on this subject; the list is a large one and it suffices to mention two items here. First, the World Health Organisation's recommendations[8] published in 1978 laying down the guidelines on which bloodtransfusion services should be based. Netherlands is a participant in this report. The second recent document is by the International Society of Bloodtransfusion concerning paediatric and exchange transfusion.[4] The report is quite clear in relation to ABO related haemolytic disease of the newborn. For exchange transfusion two lines have been recommended:

1. Group O blood with low anti + titre and haemolysins; this is the common British practice
2. Group O red cells suspended in AB plasma; this is the American practice.

We prefer to follow the second choice.

However, this does not seem to be acceptable to some of our paediatric colleagues. They wish Witebsky substance to be added to blood. What exactly is Witebsky substance? It is an animal substance (Fig. 2). It is marketed as a reagent and is not intended for intravenous use. If used intravenously as a medicament it ought to be included in the pharmacopoeias or be registered by the local drug authorities. It is not mentioned in the European, American or British pharmacopoeias or locally registered.

The American Federal Drug Authority has clearly laid down in its Regulations[2] that Witebsky-substance is not to be used intravenously. In fairness to the manufacturers, they seem to be unaware of the practice. The product literature includes the categorical statement "Not for intravenous use". If this fails the manufacturer should consider withdrawing the product from the market.

Figure 2

ANIMAL A + B SUBSTANCE

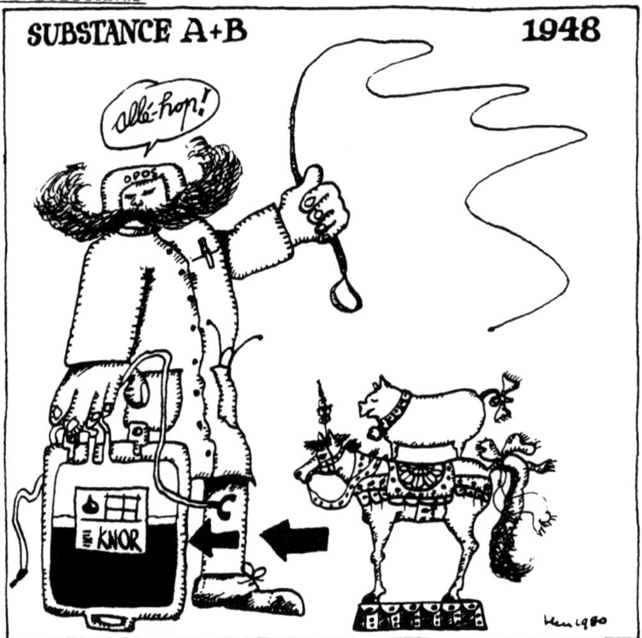

Knowing all this, why then is such an antiquated and potentially dangerous practice being demanded in the Netherlands?

Some paediatricians assume that fresh heparinised blood for every exchange transfusion is a highly desirable commodity. Not only is the assumption never to be questioned but it is reinforced by tradition. Let me demonstrate the fallacy and danger of such a practice from an actual case.

On the evening of 16 July 1980 a paediatric unit 80 km distant asked me to supply fresh heparin blood of A Rh negative, Kell negative and Jkb negative type for exchange transfusion. This was the third pregnancy for a mother whose previous history indicated that she had had this problem before. At least two weeks before delivery the mother's serum clearly demonstrated the presence of several immune antibodies corresponding to father's red cell antigens, which was already known. No attempt to arrange for compatible blood to be available had been made and we were left with this problem at the eleventh hour. The best I could do at that moment was to make 10 units of group A Rhesus negative blood not more than 48 hours old directly available from the bank for selection and cross matching. This suggestion was not accepted and twice that night we had to call in donors. Against our advice heparin blood was supplied. Following that practice, what were the chances that night of finding suitable blood (Fig.3)? From the knowledge of the blood group distribution one could definitely predict that they were slight (Table II).

Figure 3

A PUZZLE HOW MANY DONORS DO WE NEED ?

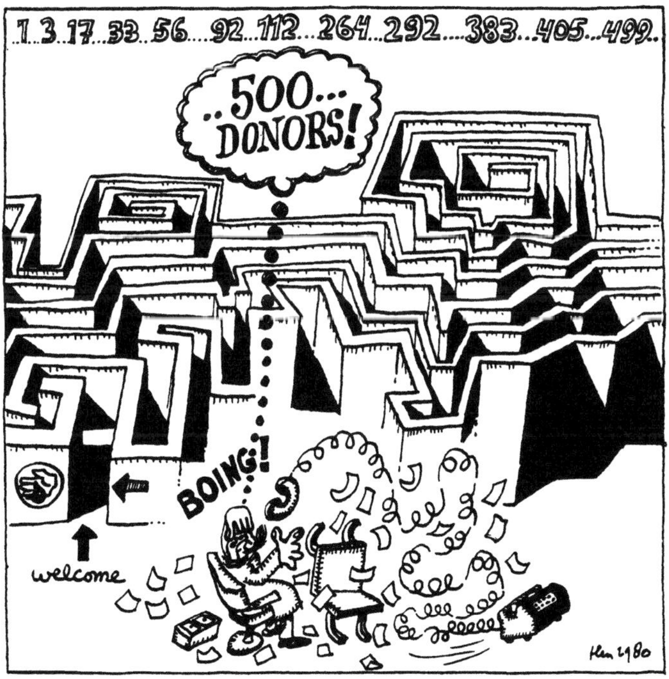

Had the mother needed blood transfusion that night it would have been a very serious situation.

For a blood transfusion, every transfusionist agrees that the blood should be cross matched. The criteria for cross matching are:

1. It should be properly done using proper media and Coomb's test. If properly carried out it should require a couple of hours. One of the pitfalls to be avoided is undue haste.
2. It should be compatible, in this case also with mother's serum.
3. In the presence of known alloantibodies it should be planned well in advance.

TABLE II

AVAILABILITY OF BLOOD

Bloodgroups	Random	Selected
group A = 42%	1:50	(A neg)
Rh neg 20%		1:5
Kidd b neg 26%		
Kell neg 90%		
Four unit:	4/200	4/20

TABLE III

CROSS MATCHING RESULTS OF FRESH HEPARIN BLOOD

Blood unit	with mother's blood
1st	Incompatible
2nd	Incompatible
3rd	Incompatible
4th	Compatible

media - saline, albumin and Coomb's test

The cross matching results (Table III) that we did the next day showed that of the four units supplied three units, as expected, were incompatible. An incompatible blood transfusion carries grave risks for the recipient, but it seems that the exchange transfusion went through with incompatible blood. Was it necessary to take such a risk? The argument is not over serology but over risk and benefit, and over the lack of forward planning and anticipation.

Lord Kelvin once said, "Measurement is an important part of scientific life". As a routine quality-control programme we measure different parameters of donated blood from the blood bag not from the pilot tube. For comparison, Table IV, derived from Geigy[3] shows blood pH values of newly born infants.

TABLE IV

BLOOD pH VALUES (38°C) OF THE NEWBORN

	mean	range
a. Umbilical artery whole blood	7.21	(7.05 - 7.38)
b. Umbilical vein, whole blood	7.32	(7.23 - 7.42)

Geigy Wissenschaftliche Tabelle

When compared with 48-hours old CPD blood and fresh heparin blood, almost all biochemical values are reasonably optimal for exchange transfusion (Table V). Our values might be at variance with the results from other sources, possibly because test samples were obtained from pilot tubes in order to preserve bag sterility. The 2,3 DPG content of 48 - 72 hrs CPD blood (Fig.4) is about 100%. Substitution of adult low affinity for fetal high affinity haemoglobin by the donor blood would cause instant rise of oxygen delivery capacity (P_{50}) in the infants.

TABLE V

QUALITY CONTROL VALUES (MEAN) OF WHOLE BLOOD

IN THE BLOODBANK GRONINGEN-DRENTHE

	CPD blood first day	CPD blood third day	Heparin blood first day
pH	7.20	7.10	7.35
Na	170	163	143
K	3.8	7.1	3.2
Ca	2.02	2.02	2.27

Na, K and Ca are expressed in SI units

Figure 4

2,3 DPG CONTENT OF STORED BLOOD.

QUALITY CONTROL STUDY IN THE BLOODBANK GRONINGEN DRENTHE

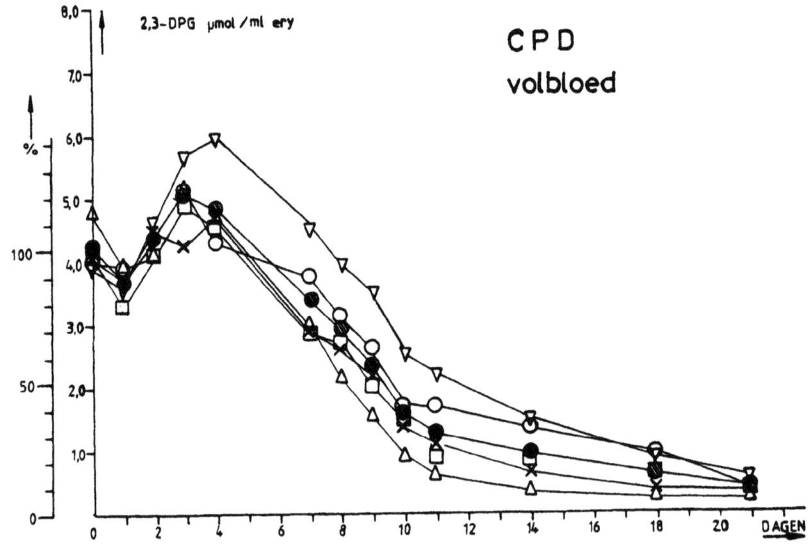

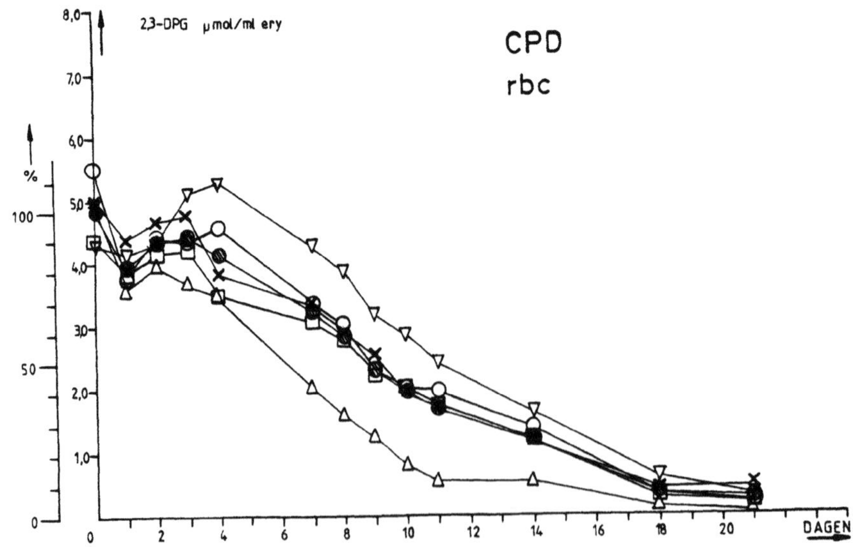

TABLE VI

BIOCHEMICAL VALUES IN CPD BLOOD:

MEANS FROM 10 UNITS OF BLOOD

	whole blood first day	whole blood 90 hours	reconstituted blood
pH	7.0	6.9	6.9
Na	170	167	168
K	3.7	9.5	9.5
Glucose	379	345	342

pH was measured on whole blood (37°C)
Na and K are expressed as millieqivalents per litre (plasma)
glucose as ml/dl (plasma)

Table according to Barnard et al[1]

In judgements made from laboratory data it is reasonable that certain kinds of evidence receive greater emphasis, and that emphasis should change as new evidence becomes available. If, solely on the basis of laboratory properties, CPD blood can be considered to carry a risk, then studies of exchange transfusion in neonates will place laboratory data in a new context. The clinical results of exchange transfusion with CPD blood as practised in some of the best centres are considerable, and are so good and gratifying that one wonders what clinical advantage can be gained using heparin blood. Additional evidence for the safety and efficacy of CPD blood in the sick infant can be found in the published literature. One such recent report comes from the combined disciplines of paediatrics and bloodbank, University of Colorado[1]. Interestingly, their laboratory data (Table VI) is very similar to our own. The clinical effects of exchange transfusion with CPD whole blood in 7 neonates were effective and optimal without any detectable evidence of adverse effects. Thus, in this context, one can rely more on data from tests in humans and less on those from the laboratory.

Recently in the Lancet[6] there appeared a review article on this subject. In relation to exchange transfusion it mentioned that in some cases this has to be done very quickly. Half an hour has been quoted. I wrote to the author, a paediatrician, inquiring how to organise and undertake this if fresh heparin blood is asked for and how to be sure that this unit will be really compatible for the exchange. She replied: "I do not have this problem; for me it is well planned, blood is already there, cross matched, reserved in advance." We support this policy (Fig.5) which begins at the early phase of pregnancy and continues through in the antenatal care to the birth of the child. If blood transfusion is necessary, with or without serological problem, then it is well planned and well thought out. Such a policy is superior to the use of heparin blood on three counts:

1. blood is already there
2. it has been previously cross matched and is compatible
3. both baby and mother are protected by this system.

Figure 5

CLINICAL BLOODTRANSFUSION POLICY IN RELATION TO PREGNANCY AND CHILDBIRTH

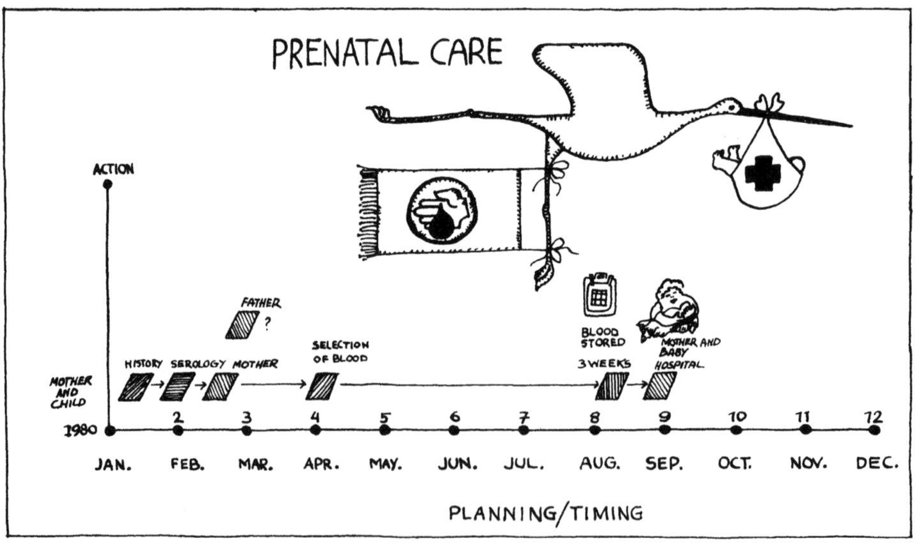

Do we then in 1980 follow recent clinical practice and scientific developments in this field, or do we go down the path with a crystal ball, guessing?

I shall finish by quoting Sir James Maxwell, the distinguished physicist known for his work on light, on how changes in scientific theories and practice come about. He said: "There are two theories of the nature of light, the corpuscle theory and the wave theory. We used to believe in the corpuscle theory, now we believe in the wave theory, because all those who believe in corpuscle theory have died."

I hope we shall be able to persuade paediatricians to change this practice in our lifetime!

Acknowledgement

My sincere thanks to my colleague, Dr. C. Th. Smit Sibinga for our stimulating discussions, to Romke Bosma, Kees van der Wisse, Dieke Bouman and Marianne Lamers, who took quality control programme as a part of the university study; to Mr R.L. McShine who stirred the serological course; to Henry de Wolf, who translated the complex medical jargon into excellent drawings, and to my secretary, Anje Luchtenberg, who typed a number of drafts and this paper.

REFERENCES

1. Barnard, .D.R., Chapman, R.G., Simmons, M.A. and W.E. Hatteway: Blood for use in exchange transfusion in the newborn. Transfusion, 20:401, 1980.

2. Food and Drug Administration, Office of Federal Register, "Blood Group Substances". Code of Federal Regulations, Title 21, Chap. 1, subpart C, 680, 20-26, 1980, p.159.

3. Geigy Scientific Tables, 7th Ed. 1970. Eds. Diem. K. and C. Lentner: J.R. Geigy, Basle, p.560.

4. International Society of Blood Transfusion: Haemolytic Disease of the Newborn: Prevention and Management. I.S.B.T., Paris, 1979.

5. Kevy, S.V.: Personal Communication, Children's Hospital Medical Center, Boston, 1980.

6. Mac Vicar and M.M. Kerr: Perinatal health and mortality. Lancet, II:1284, 1979.

7. Stathkis, N.E. and Mosseson: Interactions among heparin, cold instable globulin, and fibrinogen in formation of the heparin-precipitable fraction of plasma. J.clin.Invest. 60:855, 1977.

8. Requirements for the Collection, Processing and Quality Control of Human Blood. Wld Hlth Org. report no. 626, 1978.

----

7. DISCUSSION

moderator: J.H. RUYS

A. KLUGE (Heidelberg, Germany): Concerning the choice of treatment, I should like to draw attention to phototherapy as a prophylactic measure in ABO haemolytic disease in the early onset of icterus. By this means we were able to reduce our figures for exchange transfusions from 20 to zero in the past two years.* This success depends on early immunohaematological determination of the O against B or A incompatibility and on careful observation of these babies - nearly 15% of the newborns - to find the few who are in danger of ABO haemolytic disease. On the other hand, in deeply jaundiced newborns coming from abroad untreated, we were not able to spare exchange transfusions by phototherapy.

J.H. RUYS: In the "Manual of Neonatal Care" recently issued from the Harvard Medical School Boston Children's Hospital Medical Center about the choice of type of blood for exchange transfusions it states that heparinised blood is generally preferable. That was the view expressed by a number of the speakers to the Session. On the other hand, it may be difficult from a logistics point of view to have heparinised blood available. If the paediatrician wants to avoid citric acids in a sick baby, is it possible for the bloodbank to afford a combination of separate components, erythrocytes, thrombocytes, fresh frozen heparinised plasma, so that the problems for the bloodbank may be avoided and the paediatrician has blood without citric acids. Could that be a solution for the future?

J.G. EERNISSE (Leiden, Netherlands): As to the heparinised plasma frozen, thawed and added to the red cells, we always get some coagulation phenomenon in that plasma after thawing. There are small particles in it which should be sieved out by a transfusion filter before this plasma is added to the red cells. That is a warning, more or less.

*Kluge, A., Schmidt, W. and L. Wille: Blut, 40:361,1980.

C.Th. SMIT SIBINGA (Groningen, Netherlands): Dr. Eernisse quite rightly brings up the problem of heparinised plasma. It is well known that heparin, especially when it is added to plasma and cooled or frozen, does precipitate some of the fibrinogen monomers. This is a normal phenomenon, which was discussed years ago. The American Association of Blood Banks Technical Manual* and Standards** explicitly state that heparin is not a suitable or acceptable anticoagulant for plasma. If citrated blood is considered to be a risk, then there are two possible alternatives as mentioned earlier:

1. removing half the plasma from the unit of whole blood, thus reducing the total electrolyte load and giving a better haematocrit (Mollison).
2. Converting the CPD blood by adding heparin and calcium (Kevy).

Dr. Ruys mentioned the logistic difficulties of the problem of trying to bring in a donor in time, and at any time of the day this should certainly not be underestimated. In cases where the infant is severely diseased and where more than one antibody is involved in the haemolytic disease, it may take a considerable amount of time to find a suitable donor. Another point is the risk of infection, not being able to screen the donor blood sufficiently thoroughly for hepatitis and syphilis, nor to lower the potential risk of CMV infection, as it will if the blood can be held for 24 or 48 hours on the shelf. It is a matter of balancing the various possibilities for the benefit of the baby.

Here the benefit is in the immediate availability of quality controlled units of blood, ready for cross matching and transfusion, whatever time of the day or night.

J.G. JOLLY (India): The real demand is for red blood cells and in that context Mollison's formula has been widely accepted. Besides metabolic changes, it becomes evident that if half the plasma is removed in such a situation there is perhaps no danger. On the other hand, if separate components are used in combination there are certainly dangers to be associated with that.

There had been a number of references to the use of AB substances to neutralise some of the antibodies in the various blood groups. Because of the risk of anaphylactic shock and the risk of the very severe types of allergic reaction, this practice has been abandoned almost universally. But if some people are continuing it would be worth hearing from them because they might have some philosophy to support their advocating it.

*Technical Manual, V.W. Miller ed., A.A.B.B. Washington, 7th ed. 1977, p.42.
**Standards for Blood Banks and Transfusion Services, A.A.B.B. Washington, 9th ed. 1978, p.9.

Secondly, as far as Rh incompatibility is concerned, we are well organised to predict it. Today we talk of IgG3, IgG4 and other fractions. But are we in any way the wiser as far as the prediction of ABO incompatibility is concerned? Are ABO HDN diseases concerned in the antenatal phase? We have tests like 2-mercaptoethanol and certain others which we use to try to neutralise one of the Ig's. It might be worth canvassing opinion as to the utilisation - our use - of such tools for prediction tests in ABO compatibility and the value of some of these substances to blood to neutralise ABO antibodies.

M.M. KERR (Glasgow, Scotland): Could Dr. Roberton expand on the process of doing exchange transfusions in the sick, very tiny pre-term baby who is neither jaundiced nor has haemolytic disease? How does he decide that such a baby has severe infection? Does he wait for the blood culture result, which will take 48 hours - it certainly does in my part of the world. Does he act on a hunch? What are his indications for doing this major procedure in this tiny infant, and does he ever have any mortality?

N.R.C. ROBERTON: There are three main reasons for doing it on small babies. One is DIC, which is obvious, because the baby will be bleeding. Another - comparatively rare - is that we know that some poison is circulating, either administered accidentally or by the obstetrician with the best will in the world to do something good for the mother.

The third is infection. There are various indicators. Obviously we do not wait for the blood culture. It is a mixture of hunch, of what the white count shows, of whether we see Gram-positive cocci in the gastric aspirate. For example, we do a small number of immature babies for group B Streptococcal sepsis, which one can make a pretty clear clinical stab at diagnosing in the first six hours of life, before the blood cultures come back. In the small sick babies it is when the baby suddenly turns a bit downward, suddenly gets a bit yellow, his white cells go up to 5,000 with a left shift, and he goes hypotensive and we have a lot of things that suggest that he has gone septic.

A.S. KHALIFA (Cairo, Egypt): Dr. Roberton showed the criteria and indications for exchange transfusion at the level of bilirubin according to the weight of the baby, but he did not show criteria pertaining to the time when the patient presents and general condition. In our own centre we are setting criteria for the level of bilirubin at which we exchange children at a level of 10 on the first day for full term babies, and at a level set 2 mgs bilirubin lower for the preterm or low birthweight baby, with yet a further 2 mgs decrease if there is acidosis. For the second day the level is 14, with similar decreases if the child is low birthweight and/or acidotic. We set a level of 17 for the third day.

BO incompatibility, or BO haemolytic disease is clinically more severe than the AO haemolytic disease. Could Dr. Garratty's excellent seroimmunological studies define this, prove it or disprove it?

G. GARRATTY (Los Angeles, USA): To respond first to Dr. Roberton. It is a coincidence that I happened to be running the bloodbank at Hammersmith Hospital when he was a registrar there in paediatrics. It is quite true that we did respond as he described and bring in donors in the middle of the night. But the system is very different country to country. It so happens that at Hammersmith Hospital at that time we had Red Cross donors - the only time I know of that the Red Cross was involved in blood transfusion in England. They had some dedicated people who seemed to be extremely pleased to come in at any time of the day or night and really loved doing it. We had a list of donors that would come in and do it separate from the normal volunteer donors who came to the normal bloodtransfusion centres.

In America things are completely different. I work for the Red Cross and it is one of the blood collecting systems. In Los Angeles we bleed over 1000 donors a day at our centres. Last year we bled 400,000 and yet we still do not have enough blood for the area. They are screaming for blood all the time. At least 80% of that blood comes from mobile operations out at factories. We find it very difficult to persuade a blood donor in Los Angeles to come to the blood centre during the daytime or during a weekend and it would be extraordinarily difficult for us to get blood donors in the middle of the night. To deal with a situation such as that described by Dr. Das, a Jk^b negative donor, would be impossible for us.

In many of these circumstances in the USA there are programmes using frozen cells, which I have not heard mentioned here. This is not very much good for an emergency, but for planned transfusions in infants many of the centres prefer to use frozen blood, which seems to have very good 2,3-DPG and removes the plasma constituents. This cannot be done at many hospitals.

To respond to Dr. Khalifa's question. What he said about the 'B's is of interest. There is some suggestion in the literature and in Mollison's book that these do sometimes tend to have more severe disease. One thing of interest may be that there have been several papers in the USA showing increased incidence of ABO haemolytic disease in black individuals as compared to white individuals. So much so that the Californian State Health Department has insisted that all babies of black group O mothers are tested at birth. Some of the problems are involved in recognising jaundice in a black infant, and these infants are discharged before the ABO incompatibility is noted. Whether this relates as well to the increased numbers of 'B's seen in blacks I do not know, but I think that Dr. Khalifa is right. There is evidence in the literature that there may be an increased incidence. I would imagine from what I do know that the affinity of anti-A and anti-B are very similar and I do not know that there is any difference in terms of that theory.

C.A.HOLMAN (London, UK): To add to what Dr. Garratty was saying. The British Red Cross no longer allows its donors to be called out after 10 o'clock at night. It is exceedingly difficult to get a donor at night.

I was stung by Dr. Kerr's last remark from the platform when she said it had to be O Rhesus negative blood. In my unit we do the ABO grouping on the babies on the amniotic fluid by inhibition tests, so we almost always have the appropriate ABO blood available.

M.M. KERR (Glasgow, Scotland): Since my haematologist is not here I am not in a position to defend it, but it is his view that any blood not ready pre-delivery should be group O. If there is time then of course we get the appropriate group, and the CPD blood will be got ready for the baby. But we like to be ready for those who literally require transfusion within 20 minutes of delivery.

J.G. EERNISSE (Leiden, Netherlands): In response to Dr. Kerr, if there is no time then of course it is necessary for the paediatricians and obstetricians to work along with the bloodbank and warn the bloodbank in advance. It does not matter whether A-positive is used for an A-positive baby with an A-positive Coomb's test. What needs to be done is to give red cells, to keep the haemoglobin at some level and to remove the bilirubin - and that will be achieved. The baby's own red cells will be destroyed, but that is a continuous process. The red cells that are added will be destroyed as well. In the meantime, as long as this transfusion is in and the bilirubin is low, the baby is safe. This will allow for time to seek out the needed donor and a further exchange transfusion can then be done.

If an exchange transfusion has been given and a second transfusion is necessary, then the serum of the mother which was used for the first cross match should not be used. A fresh sample should be taken from the baby after the first transfusion. If the first donor happened to have some antibody, if the donor himself had not been screened for irregular red cell antibodies, then if an antibody is introduced there will be a haemolytic transfusion reaction after the second transfusion.

T.L. TURNER: I would support the suggestion that CPD blood has advantages, and like the majority of my British colleagues support the view that heparinised blood is unnecessary for the majority of exchange transfusions.

----

1. USE OF INFUSION PUMPS FOR PAEDIATRIC BLOOD TRANSFUSION

A.J. SMALLENBROEK, B.D.R. BOITEN and C.Th. SMIT SIBINGA

To prevent circulatory overload, infusion apparatus is generally used in paediatric practice. However, the infusion pumps that are available are not designed for the transfusion of blood and blood components. To find out whether these pumps are suitable and safe for this purpose, the three basic types of IVAC infusion apparatus in use at the University Hospital Department of Paediatrics in Groningen were investigated.

The IVAC 231 is an infusion controller driven by gravity and not an active pump. The IVAC 531 is a peristaltic pump and the IVAC 630 is a volumetric pump. Cell damage or haemolysis were studied using whole blood and red cell concentrates of 2 days shelf life.

EXPERIMENTAL SET-UP

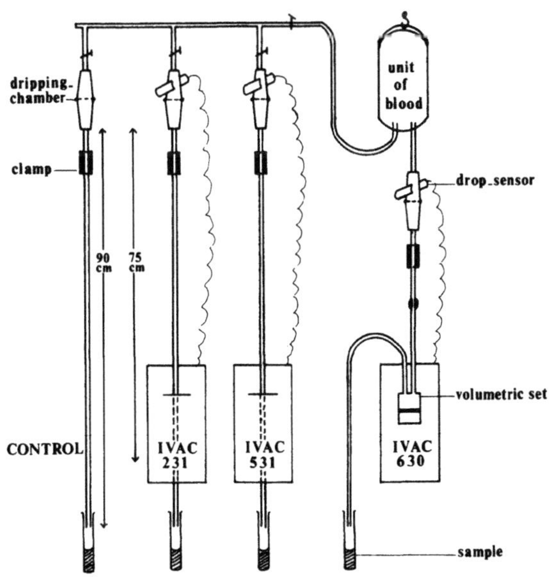

PLASMA-HAEMOGLOBIN

C=control   5, 25 resp. 60 = flow in drops/min

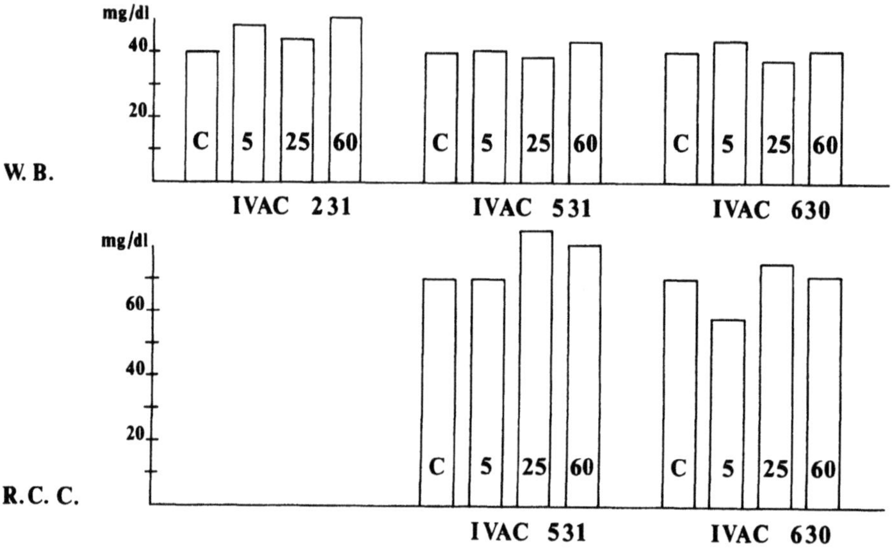

PLASMA-POTASSIUM

C= control   5, 25 resp. 60 = flow in drops/min

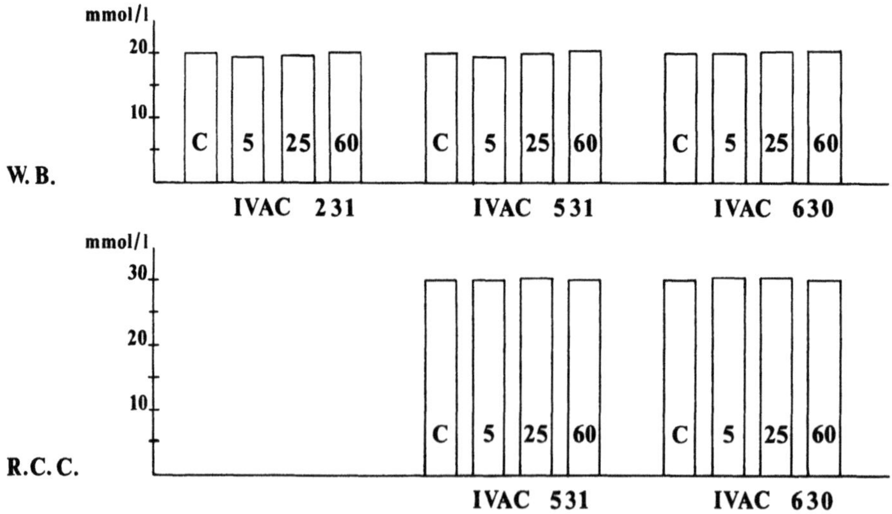

In the experimental set-up, to allow for comparisons one unit of blood was used for all three pumps running parallel with a control infusion set without a pump (Fig. 1). Samples were taken at three different flow rates:

5 drops/minute (about 15 ml/hour)
25 drops/minute (about 90 ml/hour)
60 drops/minute (about 230 ml/hour).

Thus a low, a medium and a very high flow rate were included.

A normal infusion set with a standard filter of 200 microns was used. The IVAC 630, however, has the disadvantage of requiring a special volumetric infusion set. This volumetric set has a 15 micron filter which is of no use for normal transfusion purposes. Because there is no volumetric set with a standard 200 micron blood filter available for this pump type, the standard system had to be connected to the volumetric set.

The following parameters were measured:

- plasma-haemoglobin and plasma-potassium as parameters for haemolysis;
- osmotic fragility in hypotonic saline, giving an indication for damage of the red cell membrane;
- albumin and total protein, as parameters for plasma protein absorption on the system surface;
- haematological data: haemoglobin, erythrocyte counts, haematocrit, MCV, MCH, MCHC, as a general quality control;
- microscope examinations of cell shapes of all samples were also done.

Figure 2 shows the most important results. Plasma haemoglobin levels of whole blood and red cell concentrate for each infusion system are given. No red cell concentrate data were obtained for the IVAC 231 because the viscosity of the red cell concentrate caused problems in the system. Control values are given for the purposes of comparison. Slight differences in haemoglobin levels were noted, none of them significantly differing from the control.

Plasma potassium levels of whole blood and red cell concentrates show, compared to the control, no differences for each of the different flow rates and different pump systems (Fig. 3).

The percentage of haemolysis as a function of the hypotonic saline concentration on whole blood experiments is shown in Figure 4. The four graphs (control and three IVAC systems) are completely identical. The data shown are obtained from the 25 drops/minute flow rate and show no differences to the control. The results from the other flow rates tested are identical to the one given.

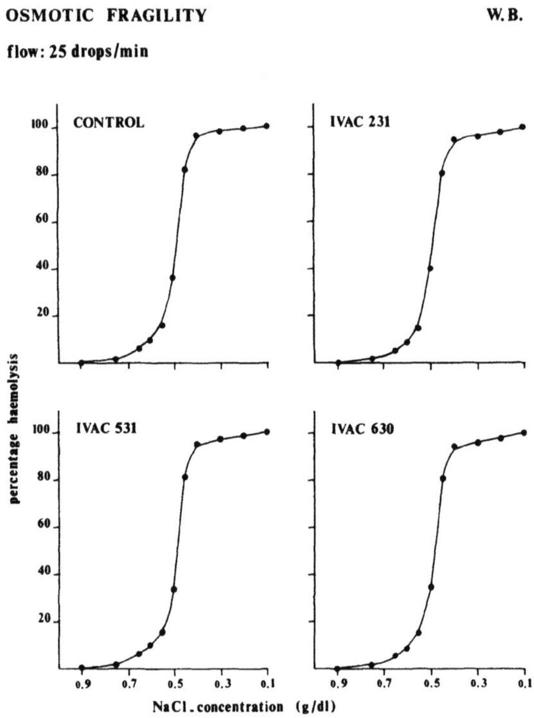

The three main haemolysis and red cell damage parameters, haemoglobin, potassium and osmotic fragility show no differences by comparison with the control system, and neither did any of the other parameters tested. Since even 21-day-old blood gave good results in the IVAC pump systems, it may be assumed that younger blood can safely be transfused using the IVAC pumps.

From these experiments it can be concluded that the three IVAC infusion systems, 231, 531 and 630 can safely be used for transfusions of whole blood and red cell concentrates. However, we noted practical problems in the behaviour of the flow in two of the three systems.

Because of viscosity there were difficulties when transfusing red cell concentrate in the IVAC 231.

The IVAC 630 proved unsuitable because:

1. So far there is no volumetric set available with the standard 200 micron blood filter. The microfilter in the IVAC set does not allow blood to be filtered through.
2. A continuous flow rate could not be obtained. The filling of the volume unit results repeatedly in a CLAMP alarm of the pump.

In summary, the IVAC 531 would seem to be the only pump that is both technically and biologically suitable for transfusion of whole blood and red cell concentrates, especially in paediatric practice.

----

2. PREVENTION OF SEVERE HAEMOLYTIC DISEASE OF THE NEWBORN BY WEEKLY SMALL-VOLUME PLASMAPHERESIS DURING PREGNANCY

J.G. EERNISSE and J. BENNEBROEK GRAVENHORST

Plasmapheresis to remove toxic substances from the circulation has become a common procedure. Paraproteins, immune complexes, toxins, lipids and antibodies are all examples of substances that plasmapheresis will remove. Industry has provided considerable help, and almost every patient on this form of treatment is hooked on to a pheresis machine.

Antibodies are also on the list. Thus it was logical to attempt to remove Rh-antibodies - although not toxic to the patient herself - by this procedure.

TABLE I

REVIEW OF PLASMAPHERESIS RESULTS

Investigator	No. of pregnancies treated	Plasmapheresis scheme	Survivals
Clarke et al 1970[2]	6	2-5 l/wk	4 (4)
Fraser et al 1976[3] (Bristol-Liverpool)	96	2-5 l/wk	59 (27)
Graham-Pole et al 1977[4]	8	14-21 l/wk	2 (0)
Pepperell & Cooper 1978[5]	3	9-12 l/wk	1 (0) (with IUT)

Table I shows that favourable results were obtained. In all these cases intensive plasmapheresis was performed with an exchange or removal of plasma ranging from 2 to as much as 21 litres/week.

A recent article by Barclay et al[1] gives details of only a single - unsuccessful - case. The authors state that failure may well have been caused by disturbance of the feedback mechanism that keeps the antibody level more or less constant. This disturbance would then cause a very strong rebound after the initial fall of the antibody level. It is this that we try to avoid by carrying out the whole plasmapheresis at a completely different level of intensity.

The system we use is not by any means our own invention. We follow the method first described by Pablo Rubinstein[6] of the New York Blood Center, and based on two observations:

- The antibody level, when measured daily with the very sensitive Auto Analyzer technique follows a peculiar pattern. During a period of about five days the level will decline gradually and then rise again sharply back to the original. It means that the same amount of antibody is produced periodically (Fig. 1).

Figure 1

DAILY DETERMINATION OF ANTIBODY LEVELS (Rubinstein, 1972)[6]

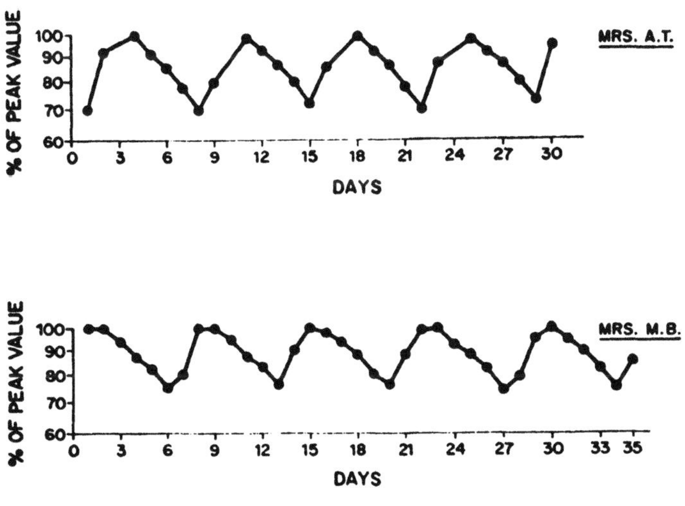

- When a small amount of antibody is removed, the pattern is maintained but the original level will not be reached (Fig. 2).

In neither case will the variations be great enough to be visible in changes of the antibody titres because this is rather a rough method of measuring the amount of antibody.

Figure 2

SCHEMATIC PRESENTATION OF ANTIBODY LEVEL DURING SMALL-VOLUME PLASMAPHERESIS

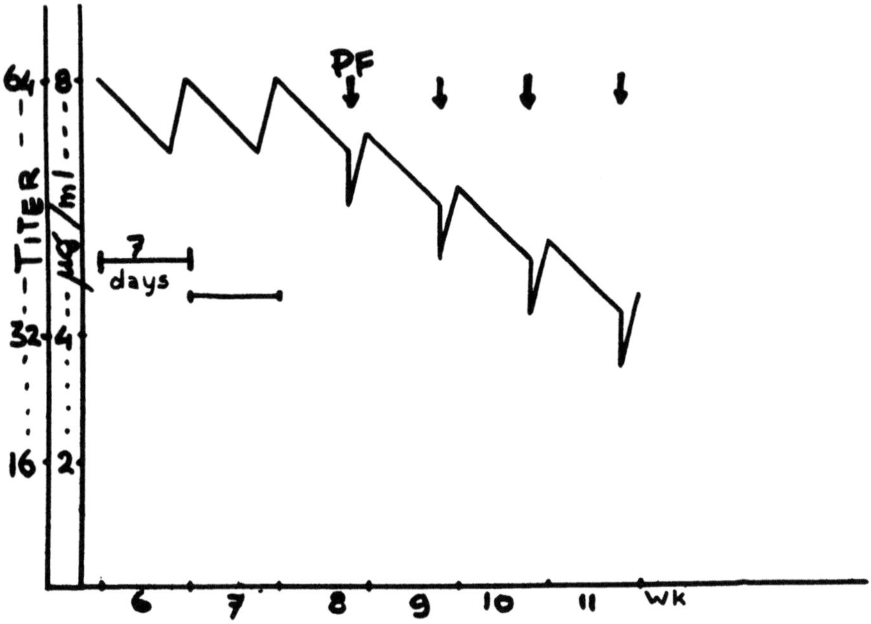

According to Rubinstein, these observations resulted in a plasmapheresis scheme in which only 500-600 ml of plasma were removed at weekly intervals and replaced by the same amount of donor plasma. Both the small amount and the time schedule were strictly adhered to in the treatment of a group of patients in Chile, all of whom had a history of haemolytic disease of the newborn. Of over a hundred pregnancies in which this pheresis scheme was followed, about 60% were reported to have ended favourably (personal communication, not yet published). Two other factors seemed to play a role:

1. treatment had to be started early, preferably not later than the 10th week of the pregnancy;
2. if the antibody level exceeded 10 μg/ml, chances were very poor.

Thus a successful plasmapheresis scheme will meet the following criteria:

- exchange of 500-600 ml plasma
- at weekly intervals
- starting in the 10th week of pregnancy at the latest.

We started pheresis according to this scheme in 1972 and since then we have treated 22 patients. All but two had a history of one or more stillbirths.

A third patient showed a sharp rise in antibody titre shortly after a bloody amniocentesis and was treated with more intensive plasmapheresis. Although she did well, she is omitted from our results (Table II). Four patients gave birth to a Rh-negative child.

TABLE II

RESULTS OF WEEKLY SMALL VOLUME PLASMAPHERESIS OF 22 PREGNANT WOMEN

LEIDEN UNIVERSITY HOSPITAL 1972-1980

		outcome	
Total number treated:	22		
Rh-negative child:	4		
	18		
		success	failure
history (no stillbirth)	2	2	-
intensive treatment	1	1	-
IN SERIES	15	9	6**

**5 hydropic and 1 dysmature

If we compare these results with those of Fraser et al[3] who published a series of 96 patients, we did not fare too badly. Quite a number of their patients had a history of no, mild or moderate haemolytic disease of the previous infant. Even then, failures could not be prevented (Table III). The numbers that really can be compared are very small (Table IV): plasmapheresis as the only treatment in patients with a severely affected or stillborn child. In this comparison our results are not at all bad. On the other hand, the intensive pheresis may have been of such assistance that an intrauterine transfusion became possible - or perhaps necessary instead of possible. At any event, in their series an IUT had to be given in 17 cases with rather good histories.

All these results point to the same conclusion, as drawn by Barclay et al[1]. By intensive plasmapheresis antibody is removed but at the cost of disturbance to a regulatory mechanism. Once this is disturbed by the removal of inhibitory factors that are present in the plasma during pregnancy, production of antibody will go on unhampered. We do not know the mechanism through which a simple procedure, such as the one we have followed, could give any result, let alone such results.

TABLE III

RESULTS OF PLASMAPHERESIS WITH OR WITHOUT IUT

Degree of HDN in previous infant	success	/total no. treated
no HDN	3	6
mild	14	19
moderate	21	32
severe (including stillbirths)	21	39
TOTAL	59	96

(Fraser et al 1976)[3]

TABLE IV

RESULTS OF PLASMAPHERESIS WITH OR WITHOUT IUT

	Leiden success	/total treated	Fraser[3] success	/total treated
PF alone	8	11	4	12
PF + IUT	1	4	17	27
TOTALS	9	15	21	39

Antibody titres certainly do not show a consistent picture (Table V). In four of the successful cases the titres remained unchanged; the other five showed a rise that was fairly great in two cases. In the unsuccessful cases the picture is hardly different. The only difference seems to be that the titres at the beginning of the treatment were higher. This was known to be a bad omen.

TABLE V

ANTI-D TITERS

Successful pregnancies PF Start	End	Failures PF Start	End
16	250	250	128*
128	128	250	250
64	250	250	250
128	128	128	500
32	64	250	128
64	64	500	500
64	64		
128	250		
128	250		

*dysmaturitas

We also looked for changes in the IgG subclasses of the Rh antibodies. None were found.

Although we do not know the mechanism through which a mitigated plasmapheresis works, we feel justified in continuing with this treatment.

CONCLUSIONS

1. Weekly plasmapheresis of 600 ml appears to improve the survival of infants severely at risk of haemolytic disease.
2. Intensive plasmapheresis of large volumes does not appear to improve the success rate of the procedure.
3. The mode of action of small-volume plasmapheresis in severe haemolytic disease remains poorly understood.

REFERENCES

1. Barclay, G.R., Ayoub Greiss, M. and S.J. Urbaniak: Adverse effect of plasma exchange on anti-D production in Rh immunisation owing to removal of inhibitory factors. Brit.med.J.280:1569,1980.
2. Clarke, C.A., Bradley, J., Elson, C.J. and W.T.A. Donohoe: Intensive plasmapheresis as a therapeutic measure in Rhesus-immunised women. Lancet, i:793, 1970.
3. Fraser, I.D., Bennet, M.O., Bothamley, J.E. and G.R. Airth: Intensive antenatal plasmapheresis in severe Rhesus isoimmunisation. Lancet, i:6, 1976.
4. Graham-Pole, J., Barr, W. and M.L.N. Willoughby: Continuous-flow plasmapheresis in the management of severe Rhesus disease. Brit.med.J. 1:1185, 1977.
5. Pepperell, R.J. and I.A. Cooper: Intense antenatal plasmapheresis in severe Rhesus isoimmunisation. J.Obstet.Gynaec.Brit.Cmwlth, 18:121, 1978.
6. Rubinstein, P.: Cyclical variations in anti-Rh titer detected by automatic quantitative hemagglutination. Vox Sang. 23:508, 1972.

----

3. INTRAUTERINE FETAL TRANSFUSION IN SEVERE RH ISOIMMUNISATION

J. BENNEBROEK GRAVENHORST and J. v. WOUDENBERG

INTRODUCTION

Intrauterine transfusion (IUT) was first reported by Liley in 1963[6]. In 1965 this method of treatment was introduced at the Department of Obstetrics and Gynaecology of the Leiden University Hospital.

During the 15 years from June 1965 to June 1980, a total of 208 IUTs were carried out in 106 fetuses severely affected by haemolytic disease. In 9 fetuses the first attempt at transfusion failed and intrauterine death precluded further attempts. Seven of these fetuses were severely hydropic. Because of the changes in diagnostic techniques and the immense progress that has been made in neonatal intensive care, it seemed appropriate to distinguish the two periods:

1. From 1.6.65 to 1.6.72
2. From 1.6.72 to 1.6.80.

MATERIALS AND METHODS

During the first period, 60 fetuses were treated with 109 transfusions. The first attempt at IUT failed in 7 of the fetuses and intrauterine death precluded any further attempt. During the second period 46 fetuses were given 99 intra uterine transfusions. Three fetuses died after a first attempt failed. Patients were selected on the basis of their past obstetric history and the results of spectrophotometric analysis of amniotic fluid for bilirubin as determined by Liley's method.[5] E_{450} values falling above the line depicting the beginning of Liley's Zone III served as the indication for intrauterine transfusion. Usually serial amniotic fluid specimens were obtained, and in most cases the decision for IUT was based on the progressive rise of E_{450} values. In the last four years, ultrasonic measurements of placental thickness and alternations in the fetal antepartem cardiotocogram (CTG) have also been taken into consideration. The intrauterine transfusions were carried out using Liley's technique.[6] The needle was introduced in the fetal peritoneal cavity under fluoroscopic visualisation.

For the past two years the procedure has been carried out under direct real time Sonography, and recently we have started using a special real time transducer. This transducer contains a slit through which the needle can be accurately guided to penetrate the fetal abdomen with the least chance of damaging vital parts. Concentrated O Rh-negative cells (Hb 16-18 mmol/l) were infused in the fetal peritoneal cavity at a speed of 70 ml/h by means of an electric pump.

The amount of packed cells infused was increased as gestation advanced from 40 ml at 24 weeks to 105 ml at 32 weeks gestation. During the transfusion, uterine activity and fetal heart rate were monitored continuously.

Usually tachycardia and a silent pattern are noticed. Bradycardia and decelerations are considered bad prognostic signs. In cases where the fetus is severely anaemic, a sinusoid CTG pattern is seen. After the blood has been absorbed from the fetal abdominal cavity, the CTG becomes normal again. Daily ultrasound measurements of the fetal abdominal circumference have proved to be a reliable means of checking blood absorption from the fetal peritoneal cavity.

After the initial transfusion, the procedure was repeated at intervals of 1-4 weeks.

Delivery was usually planned to take place 2-4 weeks after the last transfusion. The weekly interval was chosen if hydrops was present at the time of the initial transfusion, and the less frequent intervals in the absence of hydrops.

RESULTS

There were 21 survivors in the first period and 24 in the second (Tables I and II). The fetal death rate in both periods was similar: 27 of 67 in the first and 18 of 49 in the second period. The neonatal death rate fell from 25% (17 of 67) to 12% (6 of 49). In the first group two children died in their first year of life of reasons not related to haemolytic disease: one because of congenital cardiac malformation, the other other found dead in its cot. Postmortem examination revealed no pathology. One cot death occurred in the second group. The overall survival rate was 31% (21 of 67) in the first period, increasing to 49% (24 of 49) in the second period. If the babies that were hydropic at the time of the first transfusion are excluded, the survival rate was 39% (20 of 51) and 58% (21 of 36) respectively. Of the hydropic fetuses, four of a total of 30 survived in the first period and four of a total of 16 in the second.

TABLE I

RESULTS IUT

	1.6.65 to 1.6.72	1.6.72 to 1.6.80
No. of patients	67	49
No. IUT	109	99
Fetal death	27	18
Neonatal death	17	6
Infant death*	2	1
Surviving	21 (4H)	24 (4H)
Percentage surviving	31%	49%

*not related to HDN H = Hydropic

TABLE II

	1.6.65 to 1.6.72	1.6.72 to 1.6.80
Fetal deaths:		
hydropic	19	9
non hydropic	8	9
Neonatal deaths:		
hydropic	7	3
non hydropic	10	3
Infant deaths		
not related to HDN	2	1
TOTALS	46	25

Initially the diagnosis hydrops fetalis in utero was made on the basis of roentgenography and aspiration evidence of fetal ascites (radio opaque dye diffusing into a large volume of fluid during the transfusion procedure). In the last four years, ultrasonic evidence of ascites and oedema combined with increased placental thickness have been added.

The incidence of traumatic death caused by the infusion procedure has been reduced from 13% (8 of 60) to 8.5% (4 of 46).

That obstetrical management has changed during these fifteen years is reflected in the percentage of Caesarean sections, which increased from 5% during the first seven years to 36.5% of the liveborns in the last eight years.

Preterm birth within a week of the intrauterine transfusion occurred nine times in the first period but only twice in the second (Table III).

TABLE III

OBSTETRICAL MANAGEMENT

	1.6.65 to 1.6.72	1.6.72 to 1.6.80
Spontaneous	16 (9)	6 (2)
Inductions	22	14
Caesarian sections	2	11
LIVEBORN	40	30

( ) preterm delivery within one week after IUT

MATERNAL AND FETAL COMPLICATIONS

In three women there was a complication, twice a placental abruption and once a severe intrauterine infection with disseminated intravascular coagulation. All the patients recovered. At present the major risks from fetal transfusions are trauma to a placenta implanted on the anterior wall of the uterus and traumatic needling of a fetus. Sometimes fetuses die within five days of the transfusion without a traumatic lesion being present. In these cases heart failure, which is reflected in a very poor CTG, is usually the cause. Premature contractions caused by leakage of amniotic fluid between the membranes and the uterine wall can usually be effectively treated with beta-mimetic drugs.

DISCUSSION

The results of the last eight years are much better than those of the first seven-year period. The neonatal mortality rate has fallen substantially, from

25% to 12%. More experience, better equipment, more active obstetrical management and improved neonatal intensive care are the main reasons for this. Death due to fetal trauma occurred in about 10% of treated fetuses in each period.

A fetal survival rate of 49% in the last period compares favourably with reports of 36% to 46% in the literature.[1,4,8,10] The 62% survival rate reported by Bowman in 1969 is outstanding but can be partially explained by different criteria for performing intrauterine transfusions.[2]

Before 25 weeks of gestation, difficulties arise in the interpretation of assays on amniotic fluid, since the bilirubin content does not always clearly reflect the severity of haemolysis in the fetus. This, and the fact that fetal trauma plays an important part in causing death in these very small fetuses, gives us reason to agree with Whitfield that fetal transfusion is only occasionally indicated before 25 weeks.[10]

Between 33 and 35 weeks of gestation, 90% of the affected fetuses survive without intrauterine transfusion. This confirms the view that elective preterm delivery after 33 weeks of gestation is safer than intrauterine transfusion at this stage.[2,7]

The treatment of hydropic fetuses with intrauterine transfusions remains a controversial issue. Some authors report a survival rate of about 30%, which is comparable to our salvage rate of 25%.[2,4] Whether these children survive without serious long-term effects remains open to question.

The use of real time Sonography for IUT reduces the risk of fetal trauma. The results over the last four years - when we have used this new technique - show an increase in the fetal survival rate (11 of 19).

Although prophylaxis with anti (D) immunoglobulin has drastically reduced the incidence of severe Rh immunisation, it will not be able to eradicate the disease. Intra uterine transfusion will continue to be needed.

Important factors contributing to low mortality are the skill of the operator and a high standard of neonatal care. The use of intrauterine transfusion when really indicated results in a more mature baby in much better condition, requiring a shorter period of intensive care.[3] In our opinion the procedure is still a lifesaving adjunct in the treatment of severe intrauterine haemolytic disease.

REFERENCES

1. Bashore, R.A. and W. Lecky: Intra uterine fetal transfusion in management of Rh disease. Obstet. and Gynec. 38:79, 1971.

2. Bowman, J.M., Friesen, R.F., Bowman, W.D., McInnes, A.C., Barnes, P.H. and D. Grewar: Fetal transfusion in severe Rh isoimmunization. J.Amer.med.Ass. 207:1101, 1969.

3. Hamilton, E.G.: Intra uterine transfusion, safeguard or peril? Obstet. and Gynec. 50:255, 1977.

4. Holt, E.M., Boyd, I.E., Dewhurst, C.J., Murray, J., Naylor, C.H. and J.H. Smitham: Intra uterine transfusion: 101 consecutive cases treated at Queen Charlotte's Maternity Hospital. Brit.med.J. 3:39, 1973.

5. Liley, A.W.: Liquor amnii analysis in management of pregnancy complicated by Rh sensitization. Amer.J.Obstet.Gynec. 82:1359, 1961.

6. Liley, A.W.: Intra uterine transfusion of fetus in haemolytic disease. Brit.med.J. 11:1107, 1963.

7. Liley, A.W.: In: International Symposium on the Rh problem. edited Robertson, J.G. and Dambrazio, F., Annali di obstetricia e ginecologia, Special Number, p.130, 1970.

8. Palmer, A. and R.R. Gordon: A critical review of intra uterine transfusion. Brit.J.Obstet.Gynaec. 83:688, 1976.

9. Robertson, E.G., Brown, A., Ellis, M.I. and W. Walker: Intra uterine fetal transfusion in the management of severe rhesus isoimmunisation. Brit.J.Obstet.Gynaec. 83:694, 1976.

10. Whitfield, C.R., Thompson, W., Armstrong, M.J. and M.McC. Reid: Intra uterine fetal transfusion for severe rhesus haemolytic disease. J.Obstet.Gynaec.Brit.Cmwlth, 79:931, 1972.

----

4. DEVELOPMENT OF INFANTS SURVIVING INTRAUTERINE TRANSFUSIONS

J.H. RUYS

The long term effects of intrauterine transfusions (IUT) on growth and development of children who were severely affected by Rhesus (Rh) incompatibility are still of interest. In the Department of Obstetrics and Gynaecology at the University Hospital of Leiden, IUTs were started in 1965. Six years later we reported in the Dutch literature our findings on the growth and development of 13 surviving patients.[2] Our data were presented in relation to published data then available (Table I). These results are in close agreement with those in a more recent publication of Hardyment et al, 1979,[1] who presented their own series of 21 patients, together with other reports on the follow up of surviving children after IUT (Table II).

Most of the children reported on by previous authors were examined in early infancy when subtle neurodevelopmental deficits are difficult to document. Relatively few of the children had reached the ages of 8 to 12 years, old enough to demonstrate any learning problems. Moreover, these older children were managed in a time period when care of preterm infants may not have been as skilful as has been the case in more recent years.

It should be stressed that when the results of follow-up studies of infants after IUT are compared with those of a control group of siblings or low birthweight infants matched for gestational age, birthweight, maternal age and social scale, similar figures for major and minor neurological defects and for mental development have been found[2,3] (Table III).

To gain more insight into the long term effects following IUT, a questionnaire was sent to the parents of 36 patients treated between 1965 and 1979. Fifteen of them had passed their 8th birthday. Two different questionnaires were used; one for children below 3 years of age and a second for the older children. These consisted of multiple choice questions on verbal and motor development, visual and auditory disturbances, school performance and behaviour.

TABLE I

FOLLOW UP STUDIES OF SURVIVING PATIENTS TREATED WITH INTRAUTERINE TRANSFUSIONS FOR SEVERE RH DISEASE

Authors	No of Patients	Age range at Follow Up (months)	Physical Examination	Neurological Examination			Mental Development		
				normal	minor signs	major signs	normal	slight retard	severe retard
1969: Gregg & Hutchinson	15	9 - 38	14 normal growth	10	5	-	14	1	-
1970: Walker	38	1 - 46	37 normal growth 5 physical handicap	35	2	1	35	-	3
1970: Franchini c.s.	16	3 - 39	16 normal growth	12	4	-	6	9	1
1970: Cochran c.s.	41	6 - 54	34 healthy 7 physical abnormalities				36	-	5
1970: Oh c.s.	11	12 - 54		11	-	-	11	-	-
1970: Fong c.s.	16	15 - 54	15 normal growth	15	-	1	15	-	1
1971: present series	13	9 - 68	12 normal growth	12	1	-	11	2	-
TOTALS	150			87%	11%	2%	85%	8%	7%

TABLE II

FOLLOW-UP OF SURVIVING CHILDREN AFTER IUT

Author and year of publication	No of Patients	Age range at follow-up	minor CNS signs	major CNS signs	normal
1969: Gregg & Hutchinson	15	9 - 38 months	11	-	4
1970: Corston et al	23	? - 6 yrs	-	-	23
1971: Phibbs et al	24	1 - 5 yrs	4	1	19
1971: Oh et al	10	12 - 54 months	3	-	7
1971: Francini et al	16	3 - 39 months	12	1	3
1971: Penich et al	18	6 - 60 months	5	2	11
1971: Walker	38	1 - 46 months	-	3	35
1972: Girling et al	26	"at least 9 months"	2	2	22
1972: Whitfield et al	48	1 - 4 yrs	4	-	44
1973: Richings	19	"at least 4 yrs"	1	1	17
1973: Holt et al	44	3 mnths - 4 yrs	-	1	43
1975: Bowman	87	" > 18 months"	3	10	74
1975: Turner et al	44	"median age 4½ yrs"	22	-	22
1976: Beck & Winkel	17	5 - 91 months	2	-	15
1977: Present Series	21	22 mnths - 10 yrs+	6	2	13
	450 (100%)		75 (16.7)	23 (5.1)	352 (78.2)

(Hardyment et al: 1979)[1]

TABLE III

INTELLECTUAL AND ACHIEVEMENT EVALUATIONS

FOR PATIENTS AND CONTROL SUBJECTS

	Patients (N = 15)	Siblings (N = 12)	High-risk Controls (N = 14)
Intelligence quotients:			
Mean	109.3	103.8	99.2
Range	89 - 149	88 - 122	78 - 115
S.D.	15.8	11.2	9.7
Achievement:			
Reading SS			
Mean	107.5	101.1	107.4
S.D.	6.4	14.4	10.8
Arithmetic SS			
Mean	99.4	98.8	94.7
S.D.	11.8	9.7	4.1

(White et al: 1978)[3]

RESULTS

The data on those patients aged more than 4 years has been analysed. There were 29 patients in this group. Four questionnaires were not returned. The results for the other 25 patients are shown in Table IV. All the children were of normal height. Mean Standard Deviation Score (SDS) was positive and the average height of the group was about one-half of a standard deviation above the 50th centile. A visual deficiency was reported in one patient but this did not interfere with his school performance. This boy attends a normal school. Two patients have a hearing deficiency. Both make use of hearing aids and attend a school for the deaf. One is retarded in school performance.

Motor development was definitely disturbed in one patient and slightly in two others. In all three cases this was coupled with moderate to bad performance at school.

TABLE IV

FOLLOW-UP OF SURVIVING CHILDREN AFTER IUT

(age range at follow-up 4.5 - 14.75 yrs)

No of Patients	Height Deficit	Visual Deficit	Hearing Deficit	Deficit in Motor Development	Speech Deficit	Deficit in School Performance
25	-	1	2	1	1	1
	M SDS*	(no retardation)	(1 with retardation)	2 ±	2±	4±
	+ 0.45			(all with reduced school performance)	(2 with reduced school performance)	
	± 0.97					

*SDS - Standard Deviation Score

Speech development was poor in one patient who was deaf as well. It was dubious in two others. School performance was bad in one patient not yet mentioned and moderate in four of the patients already mentioned as having deficiencies in hearing, motor and speech development.

Behaviour was characterised by reduced concentration in 8 patients and restlessness in 6. The available data did not allow conclusions to be drawn about the presence of the minimal brain dysfunction syndrome.

Some patients had more than one deficiency. Of the 25 patients, 4 (16%) had definite disturbances and 4 (16%) had a non-optimal development. In comparison with other surveys and series (Table V) the conclusion emerges that with the increasing length of follow up, the frequency of major signs of disturbed development becomes higher. However, the results are not worse than those of a control group.

TABLE V

FOLLOW UP STUDIES OF SURVIVING CHILDREN AFTER IUT

Authors	No of Patients	Length of follow-up (maximum)	Normal	Minor signs	Major signs
1971: Ruys	150	5 yrs	± 85%	± 10%	± 5%
1979: Hardyment et al	450	10 yrs	± 78%	17%	5%
1979: Hardyment et al	21	10 yrs	62%	29%	10%
1980: Present series	25	14.75 yrs	68%	16%	16%

In the follow up studies reported till now, no special attention has been paid to a possible correlation between the presence of hydrops at birth and bad results at follow up. In our series of 25 patients, 5 were hydropic at birth. Three of them belong to the group of 4 patients with definite disturbances. One of them had a non-optimal development (Table VI). Therefore, we would conclude that in our series the majority of patients with developmental disturbances were hydropic at birth.

TABLE VI

PROGNOSIS AFTER HYDROPS AT BIRTH

IN SURVIVING CHILDREN

At birth		At follow-up	
		Definitely Disturbed	Non-optimal
Hydropic	5	3	1
Non-hydropic	20	1	16

CONCLUSIONS

Children who suffered from haemolytic disease of the newborn and were born after IUTs and preterm labour, particularly those hydropic at birth, who underwent exchange transfusions and possibly suffered from neonatal complications, are to be regarded as at risk of developmental disturbance.

REFERENCES

1. Hardyment, A.F., Salvador, H.S., Towell, M.E., Carpenter, C.W., Jan, J.E. and A.J. Tingle: Follow-up of intrauterine transfused surviving children. Amer.J.Obstet.Gynec. 133:235, 1979.
2. Ruys, J.H.: De behandeling van pasgeborenen met de ernstigste vormen van erythroblastosis foetalis. In: Rhesus antagonisme, De Nederlandse Bibliotheek der Geneeskunde, Stafleu, Leiden, 1971, deel 67.
3. White, C.A., Goplerud, C.P., Kisker, C.Th., Stehbens, J.A., Kitchell, M. and J.C. Taylor: Intrauterine fetal transfusion, 1965 - 1976, with an assessment of the surviving children. Amer.J.Obstet.Gynec. 130:933, 1978.

5. DISCUSSION

moderator: S.P. ISRAËLS

A.S. KHALIFA (Cairo, Egypt): Professor Bennebroek Gravenhorst has said that there is no correlation between the level of bilirubin and the severity of the clinical connection. Can he elaborate?

J. BENNEBROEK GRAVENHORST: This only applies to fetuses prior to 24 weeks of gestation. In the very early stage it is difficult to draw conclusions from the amount of bilirubin present in the amniotic fluid.

C.A.HOLMAN (London, England): Professor Bennebroek Gravenhorst mentioned the value of ultrasound. In London there is one obstetrician who uses a fetoscope with the ultrasound, and working together with him we have now transfused babies before 24 weeks intravascularly as a treatment for their hydrops. It requires a great deal of skill which this obstetrician has. It is a new development which should help to rescue these babies that hitherto have almost always died, even with intrauterine transfusion.

J.G. JOLLY (India): Professor Bennebroek Gravenhorst has rightly emphasised the importance of spectrophotometry and other investigations before taking a decision about intrauterine transfusion. Does he know of any direct correlation between indirect Coombs testing and spectrophotometric analysis that might help in taking a decision on intrauterine transfusion?

J. BENNEBROEK GRAVENHORST: The correlation is very poor and it only exists in the first pregnancy where Rhesus antibodies occur. It Rhesus antibodies already exist, it is very difficult to find a real correlation between the bilirubin content of the amniotic fluid and the concentration of antibodies in the serum.

----

1. CYTOMEGALOVIRUS INFECTIONS

A.C. HEKKER

Infection is not the same thing as disease. In an infection an organism invades the body and multiplies in it. It may be silent and cause no reaction in the body other than a rise in antibody titre and production of IgM antibodies. In disease, on the other hand, the invading organism causes damage to tissues. This may be so slight that the patient has no symptoms and the damage can be detected only by laboratory tests. Cytomegalovirus (CMV) is such an organism. Its passage through the body is most often silent.[4,7,9]

Cytomegalovirus is an ubiquitous virus. The incidence and age distribution of infection varies strikingly with socio-economic status and part of the world. In the countries of Asia and Africa more than 90% of the population become infected and acquire antibodies by 5 years of age and much of this is early perinatal and postnatal infection.

In the more developed areas of the world however, major exposure occurs in adolescence and early adult life.

After an infection the virus is isolated from urine, saliva and other excreta and also from blood. There is an antibody rise in the complement fixation test and the patient produces CMV-specific IgM antibodies. The virus stays present in the patient's leucocytes for the rest of his life. Reactivation of infection can occur and is mostly without symptoms.

Under certain circumstances primary CMV infection can be a problem or even cause serious disease:

1. In patients having undergone a bone marrow transplantation CMV is a big killer by causing interstitial pneumonia.
2. In kidney transplant recipients CMV can be the cause of a serious set-back. Even rejection of the kidney seems to be associated with an infection.
3. Post transfusion mononucleosis is caused by CMV.[2]

If we are of the opinion that in the interests of the patient the primary CMV infection must be avoided, it can be avoided.

1. On several occasions we have found that in a normal blood donor population 1-2% has a primary CMV infection. In the blood of these donors CMV-specific IgM can be detected and the virus can be isolated from urine, saliva and blood. The donors we found in this situation did not show any clinical symptom. One remembered that there had been a case of mononucleosis in his environment. It would be wise not to use their blood for transfusion, whether as fresh blood or whether after storage over a couple of days. As thermodegradation experiments with live CMV in blood have yet to be done, it is not yet known how long the virus survives. It is also not yet known how long the blood from donors with a primary CMV infection is infectious, or if the infectiousness ever disappears.
2. Do not give blood, a kidney or another organ from donors who are CMV positive (by virus isolation or antibodies) to recipients who have never had a CMV infection. Methods for rapid detection of antibodies are available.
3. There is an experimental live CMV vaccine. This vaccine deserves much more attention in the set of surgeons and clinicians who are responsible for kidney transplantation, especially in children.

CMV, like rubellavirus, destroys or severely damages fetal cells. Intrauterine CMV infection tends, therefore, to cause several congenital malformations.[1] The classical congenital "cytomegalic inclusion disease" is a serious disease and most of the infants die within a few days of birth. If they survive, serious congenital defects result.[3] If less organs are infected the symptoms are less serious and even a number of intrauterine infected children are born apparently normal.[5] As at least 1% of a normal population and therefore also of pregnant women have a primary CMV infection, 1% of pregnancies with an intrauterine infection caused by CMV can be expected. Data from several studies confirm this supposition. The number of newborns with serious congenital CMV infection however, is fortunately and, may be, surprisingly small.

The diagnosis of intrauterine CMV infection can be made by detection of CMV specific IgM in the cord blood or in babies' blood taken within 10-14 days after birth. The virus can be isolated from urine from the day of birth on. We cannot be sure from samples of serum or urine taken later than 14 days after birth that the child suffered an intrauterine infection because the child may be infected during delivery or immediately after birth.[6]

When an infant is infected during delivery (it is said that, at the end of pregnancy, at least 10% shed CMV in the cervix uteri) or the infant is infected after birth (because of cuddling by mother or aunts or because it is exsanguinated) the infection is usually silent.[8] Infants start to excrete the virus in urine and saliva and to develop CMV specific IgM in the blood not earlier than 14 days after birth. After a certain period of time the specific IgM disappears from the blood. The excretion of virus however, as in intrauterine infected children, goes on for months or even years.

TABLE I

CONGENITAL CYTOMEGALIA

Nr	Symptoms	age (days)	IgM antibodies (indirect IF)	CMV in urine and saliva on age (days)
1	congenital malformation, IgM	12	65536	12
2	microcephaly, thrombopenic purpura	2	4096	2
3	dysmature, thrombopenic purpura	1	64	14
4	microcephaly	12	512	nd
5	"intrauterine infection" IgM	6	128	nd
6	"light for dates" IgM	14	256	14
7	thrombopenic purpura	2	2048	11
8	microcephaly	4	128	nd

nd = not done

Table I shows 8 children with symptoms of congenital CMV. The children had CMV specific IgM in their blood, 5 patients were tested for virus excretion, and all 5 were found to be positive. The diagnosis could be made because samples were taken within 14 days after birth.

Table II is an example of CMV infection in 3 children in whom it is not possible to point to an intrauterine CMV infection because the serum and urine were tested too late for CMV-specific IgM and virus respectively.

The diagnosis intrauterine CMV infection canot be made solely on clinical grounds. Table III presents material from two children with symptoms suggesting intrauterine CMV infection. However, the mothers of these children never had a CMV infection in their lives.

TABLE II

CMV INFECTIONS

Nr	Symptoms	age (months)	IgM antibodies (indirect IF)	CMV in urine & saliva on age (months)
9	intracerebral calcifications, microcephaly	4	128	5
10	congenital malformation,IgM	2	512	2
11	congenital malformation in CNS	3	256	3

TABLE III

CMV INFECTION AFTER BIRTH

WITH CONGENITAL MALFORMATION OF UNKNOWN AETIOLOGY

Nr	Symptoms	age (months)	IgM antibodies (indirect IF)	CMV in urine & saliva on age (months)	compl fixing antibodi
12	premature thrombopenic purpura, bl.tr.mother 2 months after delivery	2	4096	2	-
13	microcephaly, thrombopenic purpura mother 2 months after delivery	2	2048	2	-

We tested hundreds of sera from children of 4 weeks to 6 months of age with one of the symptoms listed in Table IV for CMV-specific IgM. In all but a sample (a child with hepatosplenomegaly) no specific IgM could be detected, so these children did not suffer from a primary CMV infection. Although a number of these children may excrete CMV, the infection is over and the symptoms cannot be caused by the virus.

These symptoms excepted, a number of other abnormalities in small children can be ascribed to CMV if the laboratory only isolated CMV without testing for IgM antibodies. In fact, we are no longer interested in the virus isolation; only the specific IgM is important.

TABLE IV

hyperbilirubinaemia
hepatosplenomegaly
neonatal jaundice
prematurity

CONCLUSIONS

1. 1-2% of regular blood donors are infectious for CMV and have to be temporarily excluded.
2. Candidates for organ transplantation who never had a CMV infection in their life may not receive an organ nor blood from donors who have had a CMV infection.
3. More study has to be done on live attenuated CMV vaccine.
4. The laboratory diagnosis of primary CMV infections must be based on determination of CMV-specific IgM in the blood and not on virus isolation from urine and saliva.
5. An intrauterine CMV infection can only be made sure by testing the cord blood for CMV-specific IgM or the blood taken within 10-14 days after birth.

REFERENCES

1. Andersen, H.K., Brostrøm, K, Hansen, K.B., Leerhoy, J, Pedersen, M., Østerballe, O., Felsager, U. and S. Mogensen: A prospective study on the incidence and significance of congenital cytomegalovirus infection. Acta paediat.scand. 68:329, 1979.
2. Benson, J.W.T., Bodden, S.J. and J.O'H. Tobin: Cytomegalovirus and blood transfusion in neonates. Arch.Dis.Childh. 54:538, 1979.
3. Griffiths, P.D., Campbell-Benzie, A. and R.B. Heath: A prospective study of primary cytomegalovirus infection in pregnant women. Brit.J.Obstet.Gynaec. 87:308, 1980.
4. Michelson-Fiske, S.: Human cytomegalovirus. A review of developments between 1970 and 1976. I. Clinical developments. Biomedicine 26:16, 1977.
5. Reynolds, D.W., Stagno, S., Stubbs, K.G., Dahle, A.J., Livingston, M.M., Saxon, S.S. and Alford, C.A.: Inapparent congenital cytomegalovirus infection with elevated cord IgM levels. New Engl.J.Med. 290:291, 1974.
6. Stern, H.: Intrauterine and perinatal cytomegalovirus infections. J.antimicrob.Chemother. 5 suppl.A:81, 1979.
7. Weller, T.H.: The cytomegaloviruses: ubiquitous agents with protean clinical manifestations (second of two parts). New Engl.J.Med. 285:267, 1971.
8. Stern, H.: Cytomegalovirus infection in the neonate and its prevention. Postgrad.med.J. 53:588, 1977.
9. Cytomegalovirus Infection. Leading Article in Brit.med.J. March 1971, p.687.

----

2. SERODIAGNOSIS AND CONTROL IN VIRAL HEPATITIS

L. R. OVERBY

The early difficulties and failures to grow hepatitis viruses in tissue culture or to infect convenient and available laboratory animals emphasise the necessity for reliable immunochemical, biophysical or biochemical procedures for diagnosing the acute diseases, for detecting the presence of the viruses in biological specimens and fluids, and for serologic analyses for antibodies in serum as evidences of exposure. Viruses in serum are usually not detectable by immunologic procedures during the viraemic phase of most diseases. Diagnosis of most viral diseases is usually achieved by isolating the cytopathic agent in tissue culture from clinical specimens, or by infecting susceptible animals with specimens believed to contain the virus. Alternately, an increase in antibody titre or seroconversion during acute disease and convalescence can be diagnostic. The presence of antibody can be observed by neutralization of the infectious agent, or by immunochemical reactions with virus antigens.

Considerable progress has been achieved in controlling viral hepatitis by accurately diagnosing the diseases through sensitive and specific immunochemical serodiagnostic procedures. Major impacts have been made in post-transfusion hepatitis and the techniques developed for hepatitis B have now been adapted widely to diagnostic virology.

THE HEPATITIS VIRUSES

In hepatitis virology we now recognise three agents:

- hepatitis A,
- hepatitis B,
- hepatitis C or non-A, non-B.

The hepatitis A virus (HAV) is not a significant problem in blood and blood products, but hepatitis B (HBV) and non-A, non-B (NANB) are. The incidence of hepatitis A, hepatitis B and non-A, non-B infections can be estimated from epidemiologic studies. Several recent studies have estimated the relative frequencies of the three diseases in hospitalised patients in several countries.

The results of seven reports are summarised in Table I. It is clear that all three agents are significant health problems, and that NANB is the major problem in transfusion-associated hepatitis. The diseases are controlled through personal and public health measures to limit transmission. There is clear

TABLE I

COMPARATIVE PREVALENCE OF
HEPATITIS A, HEPATITIS B, AND NON-A,NON-B HEPATITIS

Study/Reference	Location	No	Aetiologic Distribution HAV	HBV	NANB
Acute Hepatitis Mathiesen et al[11]	Greece	216	10%	74%	16%
Acute Hepatitis Norkrans et al[16]	Sweden	480	22%	62%	13%
Acute Hepatitis Mathiesen et al[12]	Denmark	115	57%	39%	6%
Acute Hepatitis Caredda et al[4]	Italy	244	30%	52%	18%
Drug Addicts Norkrans et al[17]	Sweden	71	32%	42%	25%
Fulminant Hepatitis Mathiesen et al[13]	Denmark	22	18%	41%	27%
Post-Transfusion Aach et al[7]	USA	282	0	18%	82%

evidence that hepatitis A can be controlled partially by passive immunisation with immune serum globulin, and that hepatitis B infections can be reduced by hyperimmune specific globulin if the antibodies are administered to patients before or shortly after being exposed to the viruses. The epidemiology of the disease suggests that perhaps hepatitis C also could be impacted by passive immunisation with either hyperimmune gamma globulin or immune serum globulin. Large pools of plasma from random donors should have antibodies to the agent.

Figure 1 shows the hepatitis A virus isolated from the excreta of a person collected during the incubation phase of disease. In comparison, the hepatitis B virus appears differently in the electron microscope; it occurs in the serum during the acute phase of hepatitis and during the chronic carrier state. The hepatitis C infectious agent has not been characterised by electron microscopy.

Figure 1

ELECTRON MICROGRAPH OF HEPATITIS VIRIONS

Left: 27 nm hepatitis A virus particles isolated from human faecal extracts

Right: 42 nm hepatitis B virus (Dane particle) purified from human serum

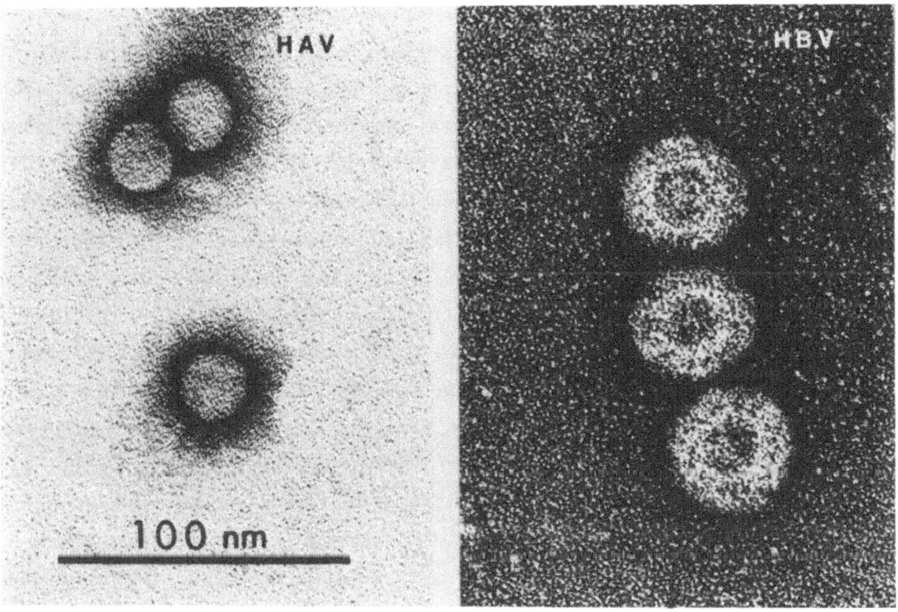

Many virus-like particles are seen frequently, but no one has clearly established a virus associated with infectivity. In due time, when large volumes of well-documented infectious plasma are available, it may be possible to isolate and characterise a candidate virus for non-A, non-B disease. None of the viruses have been well characterised classically through growth in tissue culture or infections in convenient laboratory animals. Nevertheless, we have been able to discover many of the biological features and life cycles of these agents. This represents a new dimension in virology and is related to the development of sensitive and specific immunological and immunochemical techniques, enabling us to discover much of the biology of the diseases in the natural host.

IMMUNOASSAYS

Almost all immunochemical assay techniques have been applied to the various antigenic components of the hepatitis viruses. This includes immune electron microscopy,[2] immunodiffusion,[3] and immunoelectrophoretic techniques,[7] complement fixation,[19], passive haemagglutination,[8] immune adherence agglutination,[14] enzyme immunoassays,[21] and radioimmunoassays.[9,20] Radioimmune assays are currently the most widely employed procedures because of high sensitivity, high specificity, and reproducibility.

The basic immunochemical methods are generic and, with variations, are currently used widely for the antigens and antibodies of many infectious agents and macromolecules. Figure 2 illustrates the use of a solid phase antibody, called a "capture" antibody bound to a convenient surface. The same antibody is used as a "probe" antibody, providing it has a radio- or enzyme label that distinguishes that antibody from any other immunoglobulin. The third component in the system is an antigen with multivalent antigenic sites. There are two reactions in testing for antigens. The first is called a "capture reaction" in which the antigen is reacted with the solid phase antibody. If antigen is present, it will be "captured" by the specific antibody. The second step may be called an "inquiry reaction" where one asks the question: was antigen present in the original specimen? If antigen was present it would be captured, and if it was captured it would react with the probe antibodies at available combining sites. The object then would be either radioactive or enzyme active or fluorescent active, depending upon the type of label upon the probe antibody. As indicated in Figure 2, this is a direct reaction: The count rate of the solid phase is in direct proportion to the amount of antigen in the original specimen.

Antibodies can be detected the same way with a two-step reaction, as shown in Figure 3. The solid phase has a "capture" antigen and one may use the identical "probe" antibody that was used for antigen detection. The third component in the reaction is a competitive antibody as the unknown. The procedure is a two-step reaction again:

(1) a capture where if antibody is present it will be captured by the antigen on the surface; and

(2) an inquiry using the probe antibody.

As illustrated in Figure 3 this is a competitive reaction. If antibody was present in the original specimen the solid phase antigen will bind less of the labelled probe antibody. These generic methodologies are used for the diagnostic antigen and antibody molecules of hepatitis A and hepatitis B, and

Figure 2

DIRECT RADIOMETRIC ASSAY FOR ANTIGEN

using a two-step procedure with solid phase and radiolabelled antibodies

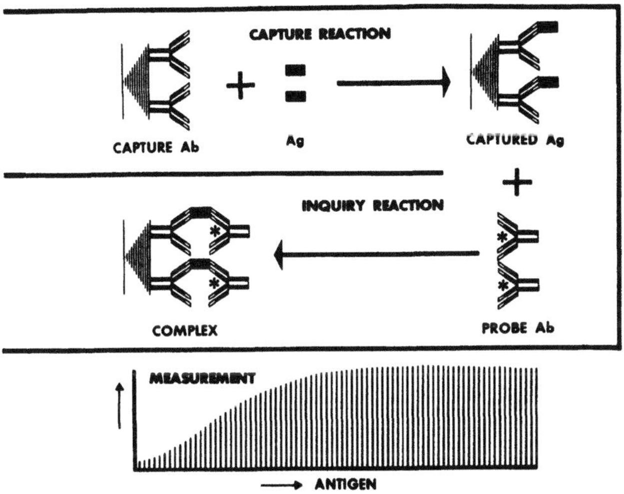

Figure 3

COMPETITIVE BINDING ASSAY FOR ANTIBODIES

using a two-step procedure with solid phase antigen and radiolabelled antibodies

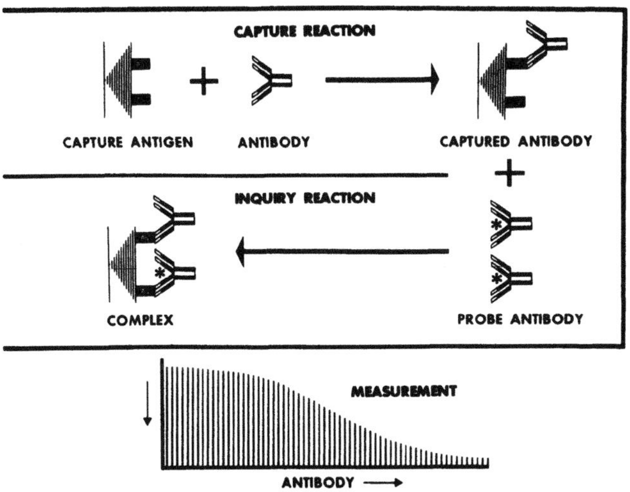

most likely, in due time, they will be used for serodiagnosing non-A, non-B hepatitis.

HEPATITIS A DIAGNOSIS

Immune electron microscopy was the first diagnostic procedure for hepatitis A antigens and antibodies.[5] The virus was obtained from faecal extracts during the incubation phase of disease. Particles were observed aggregated with antibody when tested with serum from convalescent patients. Currently, radioimmune assays or enzyme immune assays using the above described solid phase procedures are convenient, practical and commercially available. Using these assays, the sequential events during hepatitis A infection have been well defined.[6] They are illustrated in Figure 4.

Figure 4

APPEARANCE OF FAECAL ANTIGEN AND SERUM IgM AND IgG CLASS ANTIBODIES DURING HEPATITIS A

time is indicated as weeks after exposure to the virus

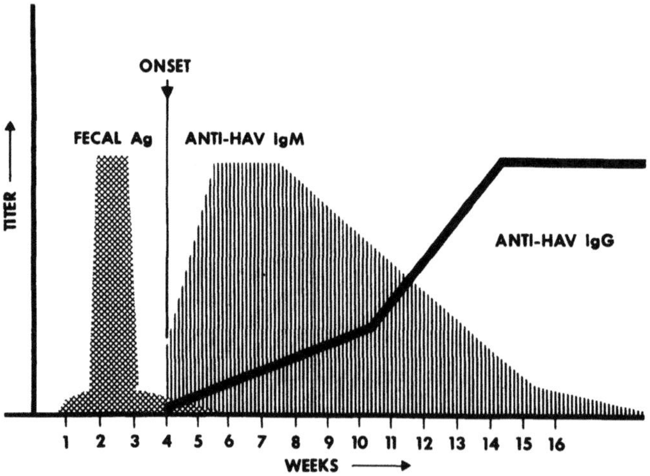

The vertical line, labelled "week 4", represents a day of onset of jaundice after exposure to the virus. The left of week 4 thus represents periods of incubation of the virus prior to the onset of clinical symptoms. The major portion of the virus is excreted in the faeces prior to the onset of jaundice. By the time of onset of clinical symptoms antibody is already present in the serum and rises in titre at a very fast rate. These diagnostic observations for hepatitis A illustrate why hepatitis A is not a problem in infectivity of blood or blood products. The virus is excreted in the faeces prior to the onset of liver disease and the life cycle of the virus in serum or plasma is very fleeting. Viraemia may occur shortly before the onset of jaundice; however, by the onset of illness specific antibody is circulating. Since humoral antibody is already present one would not expect an infectious agent in the blood at this time.

Reference to Figure 4 indicates that one could diagnose hepatitis A infection:

(1) by detecting the virus in the stool during incubation and before the onset of jaundice

(2) by a seroconversion

(3) by a rapidly increasing antibody titre on paired specimens during acute disease.

The current and more practical method to diagnose hepatitis A acute disease is to determine if the antibody to hepatitis A is an IgG or an IgM class. If it is predominantly IgM this represents acute disease. If it is exclusively IgG this signifies a persisting immunity and that the current symptoms are not due to hepatitis A infection.

HEPATITIS B DIAGNOSIS

The hepatitis B virus is a DNA virus but has some new dimensions not known in any other class of viruses. The infectious virus occurs in serum at a very low concentration and is not detectable directly by immunoassays. The defective form of the virus, HBsAg, contains only the outer shell and occurs in large quantities in serum when virus is present. HBsAg is therefore readily detectable by immunoassay. The carrier state for the hepatitis B virus is well known. In the United States it is estimated that there are 700,000 - 1,000,000 HBsAg carriers. Many of them are healthy and may participate in plasmapheresis and blood donation. They also represent a reservoir of infectious agents in the population, inducing a steady state of infectivity and new carriers. Worldwide, the number of HBV carriers is estimated to be 160 or 180 million. HBsAg screening identifies these carriers as risks for transmitting disease to close personal contacts, in plasmapheresis and in transfusion services.

The various virion components for the hepatitis B virus are illustrated in Figure 5. In addition to the intact virus several of the components are released to the serum free of the virus. The surface antigen (HBsAg) also occurs in serum as 22 nm particles without a core, possibly 100,000 to a million times more numerous than the infectious virus (HBV). The internal nucleocapsid of

Figure 5

STRUCTURE OF THE HEPATITIS B VIRUS

ILLUSTRATING THE ANTIGENIC COMPONENTS: HBsAg, HBcAg, and HBeAg

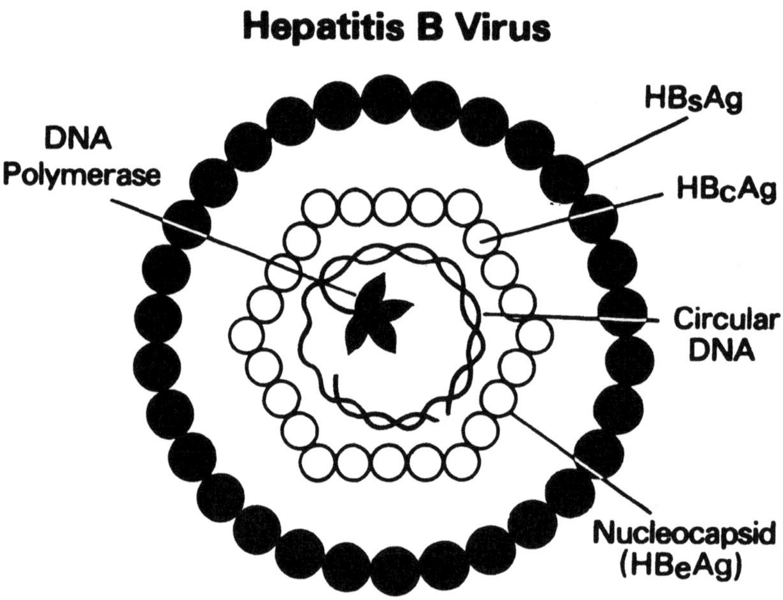

the infectious virus represents the core antigen (HBcAg).[2,18] The nucleocapsid does not occur free in serum. The e-antigen is a small molecule associated with the hepatitis B virus first reported by Magnius and Espmark.[10] It can be recognised in serum by immunodiffusion and by radioimmunoassay.[15] HBeAg occurs only in HBsAg-positive serum. It is part of the infectious virion and, like HBsAg, is produced in large excess during virus replication. The diagnostic molecules of HBV are illustrated in Figure 6. The virion components induce an immune response; therefore, the immunologic systems for hepatitis B are:

(1) the surface antigen in its antibody (Fig. 6A);

(2) the core antigen and its antibody (Fig.6 C and D); and

(3) the e-antigen and its antibody (Fig.6 E). The surface antigen is the outer shell of the virus. The core antigen is the nucleocapsid, and the e-antigen is associated in an unknown way with the infectious virus. The surface antigen and the e-antigen occur in many thousandfold excess over the virus particles. They are therefore easy to detect in plasma. Large quantities of DNA are also frequently found in serum containing HBsAg (Fig.6 F). The diagnostic significance of this nucleic acid is unknown.

Figure 6

HEPATITIS B COMPONENTS FOUND IN SERUM AND LIVER

A. 22 nm HBsAg particles

B. Filamentous HBsAg particles

C. Complete virions (Dane particles)

D. Nucleocapsid core particles from hepatocyte nuclei

E. Immunodiffusion pattern illustrating HBsAg in peripheral wells and HBeAg in wells 2 and 4

F. Circular DNA from Dane particles

G. Linear DNA from HBsAg-positive serum

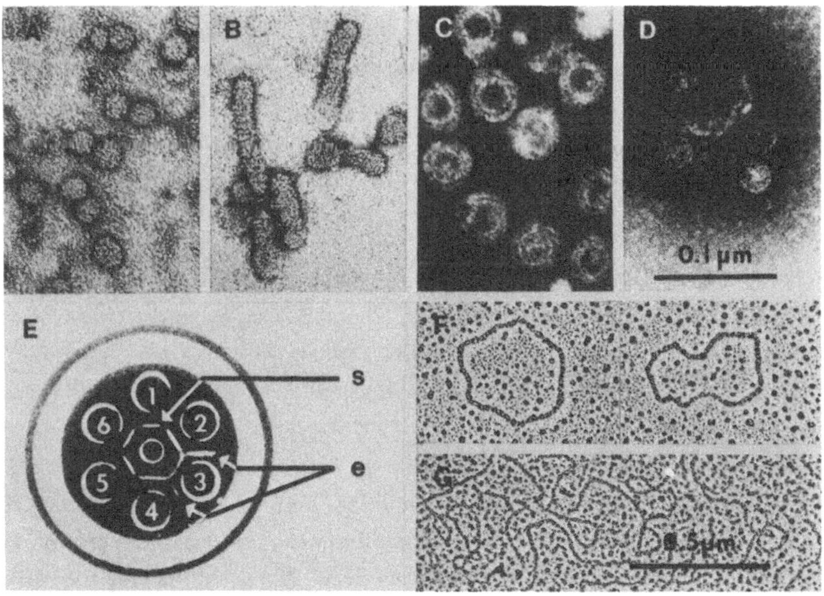

During the course of infection the antigenic components of the hepatitis B virus appear in serum, and antibodies arise. With the six tests for the diagnostic molecules available their sequential rises and falls may be outlined.

Figure 7

ILLUSTRATION OF THE SEQUENTIAL APPEARANCE OF HEPATITIS B VIRUS ANTIGENS AND ANTIBODIES IN SERUM THROUGHOUT THE ACUTE DISEASE, CONVALESCENCE, RECOVERY AND IMMUNITY PHASES OF INFECTION

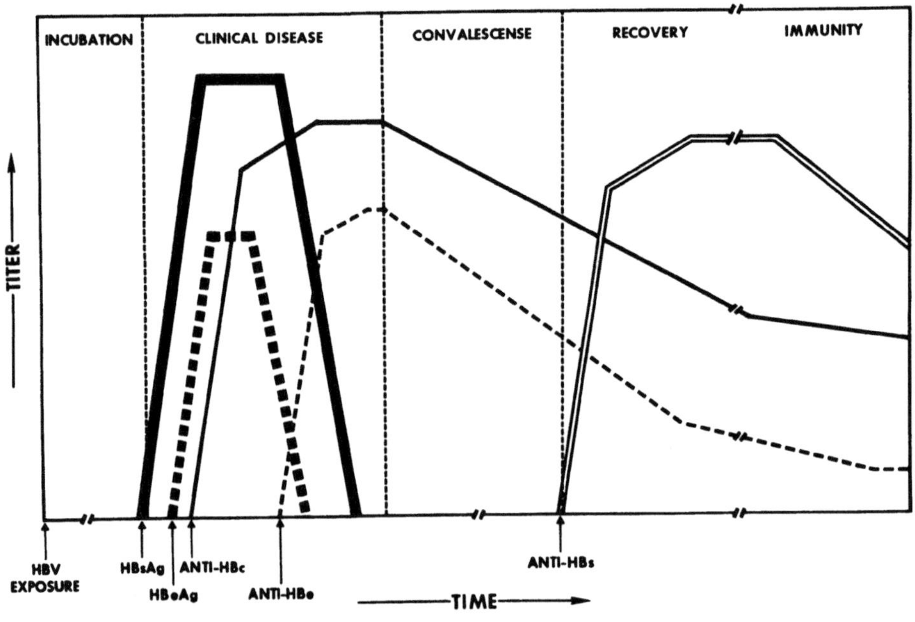

The general scheme is shown in Figure 7. When only the surface antigen is positive and all of the others are negative, this signifies an early phase of virus replication after a period of incubation. When the surface antigen and e-antigen are positive, this represents increasing viral replication and perhaps the onset of clinical symptoms. If we find surface antigen, anti-core, and e-antigen positive, this represents the peak of viral replication and the peak of increasing clinical symptoms. The presence of anti-core, anti-e and surface antigen represents the resolution of viral replication, the onset of resolution of disease, and a decreasing titre of surface antigen. If two antibodies are positive (anti-core and anti-e), this represents a period of convalescence where the surface antigen is below detectable levels. During the immunologic responses to the hepatitis B virus there is a convalescing period when both surface antigen and its antibodies are undetectable. Anti-core and anti-e are markers for this period. Finally, if three antibodies are positive (anti-core, anti-e and anti-surface), this represents a period of recovery and persisting immunity. Throughout the period of contact with the virus (incubation, acute disease, convalescence and recovery), only the last period suggests an absence for the hepatitis B virus in either a free or immune complex form.

HEPATITIS B CARRIERS

The above discussion has dealt with acute disease, convalescence and recovery. There are two other situations that occur frequently after hepatitis B infection. A state may result where the surface antigen continues positive for a long time, perhaps years or a lifetime. Anti-core and e-antigen also persist. The persistence of these markers suggests that viral replication continues and the risk of infectivity and chronic disease would be very high. There are exceptions but the generality for infectivity and poor prognosis appears convincing.

Alternate form of persisting viral antigenaemia is reflected by e-antigen seroconversion to anti-e. The persistence of anti-core and anti-e represents a low level of virus replication. This serology correlates with the healthy carrier state, low infectivity and good prognosis. There are exceptions and the correlations are not absolute.

Screening for HBsAg is a valuable aid in identifying HBV carriers and reducing transfusion and blood products-associated hepatitis B. A profile of all of the serologic markers of the virus is a valuable diagnostic aid in patient care, for epidemiology and for prognostic implications during the carrier state.

TRANSFUSION ASSOCIATED HEPATITIS

Despite wide scale screening of donor blood for HBsAg by increasingly more sensitive tests, transfusion-associated hepatitis still remains an important health problem. With third generation screening of blood and blood products, selection of blood donors, and a general awareness of the epidemiology of hepatitis B we can estimate that B type hepatitis associated with transfusion has been reduced up to 80%. The exact incidences before and after the introduction of screening are difficult to obtain. An estimate of the changing incidences of post-transfusion hepatitis in North America and Western Europe is illustrated in Figure 8.

Figure 8

ILLUSTRATION OF THE RELATIVE INCIDENCE OF

TRANSFUSION-ASSOCIATED VIRAL HEPATITIS

BEFORE AND AFTER INTRODUCTION OF SCREENING OF BLOOD DONORS FOR HBsAg

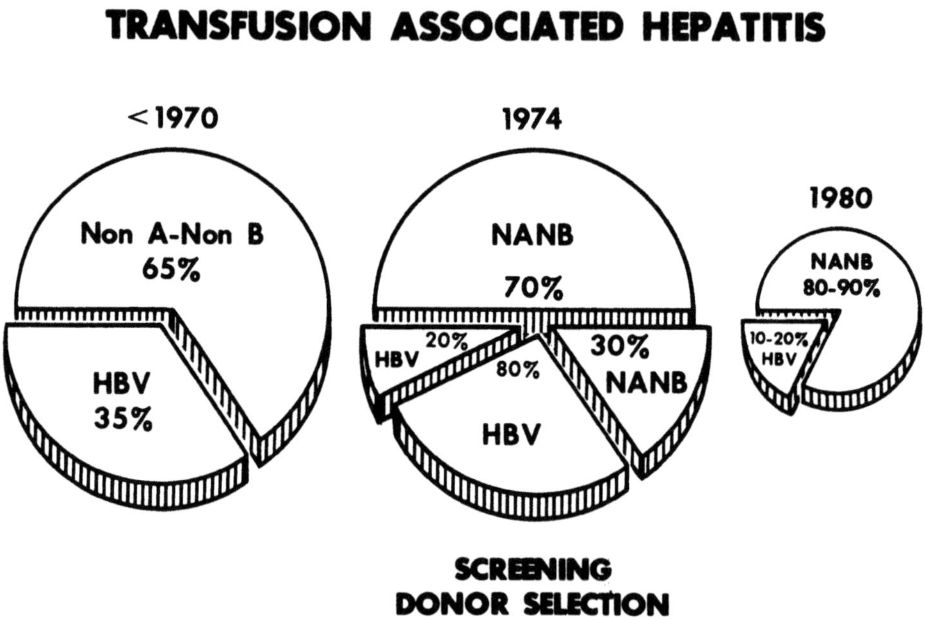

Prior to introduction of "third generation" screening and donor selection in 1974, B type hepatitis represented about 30–40% of the total. Some exposure to B type hepatitis remains even after careful donor selection and blood positive by third generation tests is interdicted. Figure 8 illustrates that total post-transfusion hepatitis has been reduced up to 50% and that the current major problem is not B and neither is it A, but it is non–A, non–B hepatitis. Of the total transfusion associated hepatitis in North America, 10–20% is B type and 80–90% is non–A,non–B (Table I).

What can we do about the B–type hepatitis that remains after third generation HBsAg screening of donor blood? This remaining infectivity could be related to donors that are "silent carriers" of HBV. One example could be a carrier where HBs antigen is too low to detect by the most sensitive tests. Alternately, there could be immune complexes of the surface antigen making it undetectable. That might be the case during the "convelescing window", a long period during recovery where surface antigen becomes undetectable and before anti-surface is produced in excess. The period can be as short as a week and as long as a year or more. In both of these cases, low levels of infectious virus could still be present in the absence of detectable HBsAg.

Sensitive radioimmunoassays can detect one nanogram of surface antigen in a millilitre of plasma. The theoretical limit of sensitivity is about 0.1 ng/ml. One ng of HBsAg represents about 10^8 particles. Therefore, when a sensitive immunochemical test is negative, there could still be a large number of particles present. Further increases in sensitivity of HBsAg tests could possibly lead to detecting additional infectious blood donors. However, a more fruitful approach may lie in detecting other serologic markers of HBV. Anti-HBc is a leading candidate for identifying "silent carriers". Reference to Figure 7 indicates that it arises early during antigenaemia and persists during convalescence and recovery.

NON-A, NON-B HEPATITIS

Reference to Figure 8 indicates that non-B hepatitis is an important problem in transfusion-associated viral hepatitis and for blood products prepared from plasma pools. Non-A, non-B hepatitis can be diagnosed by exclusion of serodiagnostic markers of both hepatitis A and hepatitis B. During acute disease episodes this would be an absence of anti-HAV IgM for hepatitis A, and an absence of HBsAg, anti-HBc, HBeAg and anti-HBe for hepatitis B. A direct serological test for non-A, non-B hepatitis is not yet available, although considerable progress is being made. Serial serum specimens from transfusion recipients during the course of disease and recovery are excellent specimens for searching for antigen-antibody systems. Although it is relatively insensitive, agar gel diffusion is a useful procedure for such studies because specificity can be assessed through lines of identity.

Figure 9 illustrates an example of transfusion-associated hepatitis with no serological markers for type A or type B disease. When the various sequential sera were tested against each other in immunodiffusion the indicated serum at about two weeks after transfusion reacted strongly with a convalescent serum taken at week 40. Convalescent sera at weeks 28 and 100 reacted weakly as antibodies.

Figure 9

OCCURRENCES OF ANTIGENS AND ANTIBODIES DETECTABLE BY AGAR GEL DIFFUSION IN A PATIENT WITH TRANSFUSION-ASSOCIATED NON-A,NON-B HEPATITIS

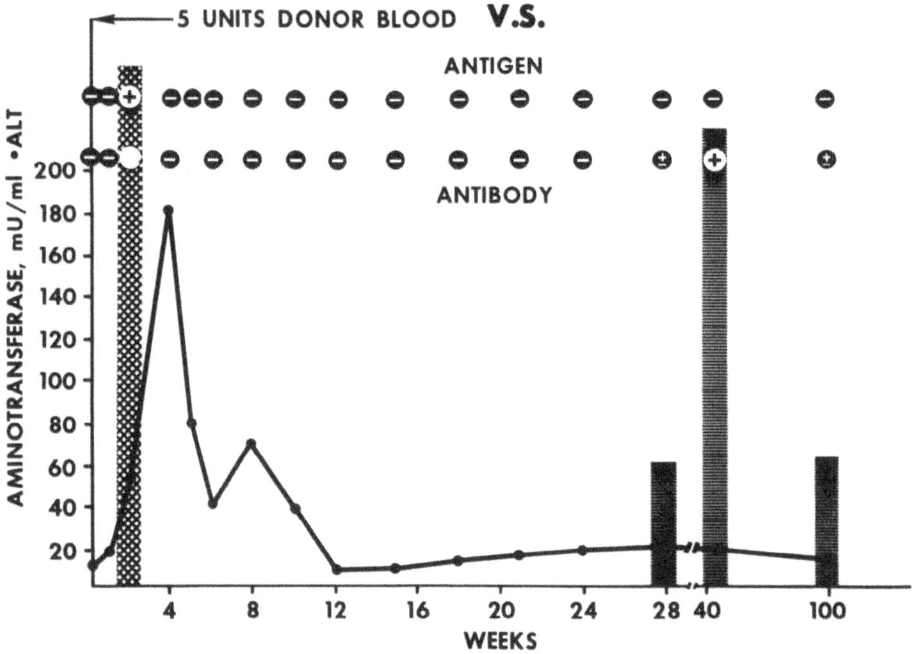

The above reactions cannot be demonstrated always in non-A, non-B hepatitis but they occur frequently and this suggests that there is an antigen-antibody system associated with the disease. If these reactions can be shown to be specific or associated with the infectious agent they could lead, in due time, to useful serodiagnostics for non-A, non-B hepatitis, following the course already charted by the many developments in the serodiagnosis of hepatitis B from the discovery of Australia antigen to the current knowledge fifteen years later.

REFERENCES

1. Aach, R.D. and R.A. Kahn: Post-transfusion hepatitis: current perspectives. Ann.int.Med. 92:539, 1980.
2. Almeida, J.D., Rubenstein, D. and E.J. Stott: New antigen-antibody system in Australia antigen-positive hepatitis. Lancet 2:1224, 1971.
3. Blumberg, B.S. and N.M. Riddle: Inherited antigenic differences in human serum beta lipoproteins. A second antiserum. J.clin.Invest. 42:867, 1963.
4. Caredda, F., D'Arminio Montforte, A., Lopez, S., Culraro, D. and M. Moroni: Epidemiology of non-A, non-B hepatitis. Lancet 2:1380, 1979.
5. Feinstone, S.M., Kapikian, A.Z. and R.H. Purcell: Hepatitis A: Detection by immune electron microscopy of a viruslike antigen associated with acute illness. Science 182:1026, 1973.
6. Frosner, G.G., Overby, L.R., Flehmig, B., Gerth, H.-J., Haas, H., Decker, R., Ling, C.-M., Zuckerman, A.J. and H.-R. Frosner: Sero-epidemiological investigation of patients and family contacts in an epidemic of hepatitis A. J.med.Virol. 1:163, 1977.
7. Gocke, D.J. and C. Howe: Rapid detection of Australia antigen by counterelectrophoresis. J.Immunol. 104:1031, 1970.
8. Hirata, A.A., Emerick, A.J. and W.F. Boley: Hepatitis B virus antigen detection by reverse passive haemagglutination. Proc.Soc.exp.Biol.(N.Y.) 143:761, 1973.
9. Ling, C.-M. and L.R. Overby: Prevalence of hepatitis B virus antigen as revealed by direct radioimmune assay with 125I-antibody. J.Immunol. 109:834, 1972.
10. Magnius, L.O. and J.A. Espmark: New specificities in Australia antigen positive sera distinct from LeBouvier determinants. J.Immunol. 109:1017, 1972.
11. Mathiesen, L.R., Papaevangelou, G., Purcell, R.H., Grammatikopoulos, D., Contoyannis, P. and D. Wong: Etiological characterization of hepatitis B surface antigen-negative hepatitis among adult patients in Athens, Greece. J.clin.Microbiol. 11:297, 1980.
12. Mathiesen, L.R., Skinhoj, P., Hardt, F., Nielsen, J.O., Sloth, K., Zoffmann, H., Moller, A.M., Wong, D., Purcell, R.H. & The Copenhagen Hepatitis Acuta Programme: Epidemiology and clinical characteristics of acute hepatitis types A, B, and non-A non-B. Scand.J.infect.Dis. 14:849, 1979.
13. Mathiesen, L.R., Skinhoj, P., Nielsen, J.O., Purcell, R.H., Wong, D. and L.R. Ranek: Hepatitis type A, B, and non-A non-B in fulminant hepatitis. Gut 21:72, 1980.

14. Mayumi, M., Okochi, K. and K. Nishioka: Detection of Australia antigen by means of immune adherence hemagglutination test. Vox Sang. 20:178,1971.

15. Mushahwar, I.K., Overby, L.R., Frosner, G., Deinhardt, F. and C.-M. Ling: Prevalence of hepatitis B e-antigen and its antibody as directed by radioimmunoassays. J.med.Virol. 2:77, 1978.

16. Norkrans, G., Frosner, G., Hermodsson, S. and S. Iwarson: Clinical epidemiological and prognostic aspects of hepatitis "non-A non-B" - a comparison with hepatitis A and B. Scand.J.infect.Dis.11:259,1979.

17. Norkrans, G., Frosner, G., Hermodsson, S. and S. Iwarson: Multiple hepatitis attacks in drug addicts. JAMA 243:1056, 1980.

18. Overby, L.R. and C.-M. Ling: Radioimmune assay for anti-core as evidence for exposure to hepatitis B virus. Rush-Presbyterian-St.Lukes med.Bull. 15:83, 1976.

19. Purcell, R.H., Holland, P.V., Walsh, T.H., Wong, D.C., Murrow, A.G. and R.M. Chanock: A complement-fixation test for measuring Australia antigen and antibody. J.infect.Dis. 120:383, 1969.

20. Walsh, J.H., Yalow, R. and S.A. Berson: Detection of Australia antigen and antibody by means of radioimmunoassay techniques. J.infect.Dis. 121:550, 1970.

21. Walters, G., Kuijpers, L.P., Kacaki, J. and H.W. Schuurs: Enzyme-linked immunosorbent assay for hepatitis B surface antigen. J.infect.Dis. 135:S311, 1977.

----

3. DISCUSSION

moderator: S.P. ISRAËLS

A.S. KHALIFA (Cairo, Egypt): I should like to stress the point on hepatitis-associated disease not only in the cases of blood transfusion but also of the component transfused, particularly for haemophilia. This really raises the question of the preference for cryoprecipitate in those patients who need it over Factor VIII concentrate manufactured commercially, because the fear of hepatitis is more in those receiving manufactured Factor VIII than in those receiving cryoprecipitate.

B. HOUWEN (Groningen, Netherlands): I would support Dr. Overby's view that IgM anti-core is probably a marker of active viral replication. In a longtitudinal study carried out in Groningen some two or three years ago, haemodialysis and non-haemodialysis patients were followed up after hepatitis B infection. It could be shown that the persistence of IgM anti-core was associated with the persistence of hepatitis B virus. In all patients who cleared the virus the IgM anti-core also disappeared.

E.E. REERINK-BRONGERS (Amsterdam, Netherlands): What are the prospects of our soon getting an easy-to-use kit for the determination of IgM anti-core? At the moment, at least for us, it is a rather laborious procedure.

In one of his illustrations, Dr. Overby differentiated between non-A, non-B hepatitis and hepatitis C. How is such differentiation made?

L.R. OVERBY: I do not know when commercial reagents for anti-core IgM will be available, but it is unlikely to be before the useful potential of such a reagent is well established. In our own laboratories we are trying to assess the significance of anti-core IgM, as is done in a number of studies elsewhere too. I believe that our findings concur with those reported from Europe that active viral replication, that is active hepatitis B virus replication, is really indicated by an anti-core IgM. It is not known up to now whether that is always the case, and whether there can be a very long persistence of this antibody well after the active viral replication is over. We are attempting the develop the answers.

Right now people are simply calling the disease that is clinically diagnosed as viral hepatitis, and where there is no marker for hepatitis A or for hepatitis B active disease, non-A, non-B. A number of laboratories are working with infectious agents in chimpanzees and everybody seems to be working with the same agent. There have been exchanges of infectious material, and if that agent is ever identified it might well be called the hepatitis C virus. Some of us are already starting to use the term hepatitis C for that agent but whether there is more than C or not I do not know. I personally believe that when we, or somebody identifies this agent that everybody is working with now it will account for the major part of transfusion-associated non-A, non-B in the US and in Europe.

N.R.C. ROBERTON (Cambridge, England): How much perinatally acquired CMV does Dr. Hekker find is due to the paediatrician doing exchange transfusions with contaminated blood or giving the premature baby a top-up transfusion with contaminated blood?

A.C. HEKKER: I do not know.

B. HOUWEN (Grongingen, Netherlands): Does Dr. Hekker believe that infusion or injection of antibodies directed against CMV would be helpful either in prevention of the disease or in treatment of present viral infection?

A.C. HEKKER: Antibodies do not even help in the person who is infected. I do not think that antibodies will help here in preventing cytomegalovirus infection.

J.G. EERNISSE (Leiden, Netherlands): Dr. Hekker mentioned that donors should be screened. How? We have one screening for syphilis, usually composed of four or five tests. We have the HBsAg test and we are to have the anti-core added.

A.C. HEKKER: You will have to have a test for CMV antibodies. There is a test available.

J.G. EERNISSE: If a donor is negative, and it will probably take some time to do the tests and have the answers back again, is that donor to be kept apart for transplant patients, bone marrow or kidney? How can one be sure that this donor will still be all right if he is needed at a given moment?

A.C. HEKKER: I know it is difficult, but it is certainly wrong to transfuse CMV into a kidney transplant patient or any patient under immunosuppression.

J.G. EERNISSE: I fully agree. As far as I know about 55% of the donors will have antibodies, and probably 55% of the patients too. It may be a bit lower in the younger age groups but it will be somewhere around that figure. Will the positives be infected or reinfected from the virus they are carrying themselves? If so, then quite a number of patients can be excluded and it will not be necessary to take precautions.

A.C. HEKKER: A primary infection in kidney transplantation means a serious CMV infection. When patients have antibodies and these are transplanted the disease is much less serious and may even be without symptoms.

P.C. DAS (Groningen, Netherlands): We have heard nothing about vaccination against hepatitis B. Perhaps Dr. Overby might give a brief resume of the situation in respect of hepatitis vaccine.

L.R. OVERBY: In several parts of the world, B type vaccines are being developed: by Merck in the United States, by the Pasteur Institute in France and by some part of the Health Service in Japan. In October 1980 I heard publicly that the United States vaccine has been in clinical efficacy trials. It was shown to be very effective in that all those people who developed detectable antibody titres were also immune during the observed period, while in the control group there have been the expected number of infections. So it is my understanding that the B type vaccine should be available on a limited basis in another year or two.

A vaccine? I believe that the virus will follow the classic enterovirus type epidemiology for immunisation. It is a question of being able to grow it in tissue culture and develop either an attenuated or a killed vaccine. I know that progress is now being made along those lines, and in the next few years hepatitis A should follow the usual pattern for immunisation.

----

1. SOME ASPECTS OF NEONATAL THROMBOCYTOPENIA

R.P.G.M. BIJLMER

INTRODUCTION

Normal neonatal haemostasis is dependent on three interrelated factors: the vascular walls, the clotting proteins and the platelets. Impairment of one of these haemostatic components may lead to serious haemorrhage. The newborn, and especially the premature, is particularly susceptible to both haemorrhagic and thrombotic tendencies because of a physiological deficiency of platelet function, some coagulation factors and anticoagulants.

Bleeding tendencies are often seen in neonatal intensive care units and are mostly associated with acute and life-threatening respiratory, infectious or metabolic disorders. Thrombocytopenia is commonly found in sick newborn infants but may be seen in the healthy newborn infant as well. There are many causes of neonatal thrombocytopenia, but this paper will only discuss some aspects of the more common ones.

Two groups of thrombocytopenic neonates can be distinguished: the healthy neonate with primary thrombocytopenia and the sick, often premature, neonate whose thrombocytopenia is only a part of his disease.

NORMAL NEONATAL HAEMOSTASIS (Table I)

Capillary fragility is normal in the term infant but increased in small premature infants.[6] Decreased levels are found for the vitamin K dependent clotting factors II, VII, IX and X, especially in the premature infant,[6,17] and for factors XI, XII[21,36] and XIII,[19] both in premature and term infants. Fibrinogen levels are normal.[38]

Levels of factor V are normal in the term infant but may be slightly decreased in the premature infant,[17,24,38], whereas levels of factor VIII are normal in the premature infant but significantly increased in terms infants.[22,38]

These deficiencies are responsible for the prolongation of prothrombin time (PT) and partial thromboplastin time (PTT) found in premature and fullterm infants. Antiproteases such as plasminogen, antithrombin III and anti activated X and XI are reduced[12,30] although overall fibrinolytic activity is normal except in sick premature infants.

TABLE I

NORMAL NEONATAL HAEMOSTASIS

Coagulation Factors	Term Infant	Premature Infant
fibrinogen	normal	normal
II, VII, IX, X	I	I I
XI, XII, XIII	I	I
V	normal	± I
VIII	↑	normal
Antiproteases	I	I
Platelet counts	normal	normal

In platelet function tests abnormalities, such as impairment of platelet retention, aggregation with ADP, epinephrine, collagen and thrombin, and impairment of clot retraction, may be found.[6,23,33] Release of platelet factor 3 may be decreased. Different findings have been reported about total platelet levels and release of serotinin, endogenous ADP and total adenine nucleotides[33,42,46,47] suggesting different possible mechanisms for the functional platelet defects in newborn infants: release defect or storage pool defect. However, these abnormalities seem to be of little clinical importance in the healthy newborn because of their transient character and a normal bleeding time in the full term and premature infant.[28] Platelet counts in healthy full term infants are in the same range as normal older infants and adults, ranging from 150,000 - 400,000 per µl. Although earlier reports[32] have mentioned much lower platelet counts in premature infants, suggesting "physiological thrombocytopenia of the premature", many other reports have mentioned normal[14,17] or slightly lower counts in premature infants.[1,3,13] Studies of gestationally classified infants found no difference in platelet counts in normal infants between 27 and 40 weeks of gestational age.[38]

Although these findings suggest that a platelet count below 150,000 per µl is abnormal and requires explanation, there is general agreement that platelet counts below 100,000 per µl are definitely abnormal.

PATHOGENESIS OF THROMBOCYTOPENIA

There is a constant balance between platelet production in the bone marrow by the megakaryocytes and destruction in the reticuloendothelial system of the liver and spleen. Normal survival time of platelets is about 10 days. Thrombocytopenia may be the result of a decreased production of platelets, increased destruction of platelets, or a combination of the two. (Table II)

TABLE II

AETIOLOGY OF NEONATAL THROMBOCYTOPENIA

1. Increased destruction of platelets
   a. maternal antibodies (isoimmune, autoimmune, drug induced)
   b. giant haemangioma
   c. disseminated intravascular coagulation
   d. exchange transfusion
2. Decreased production of platelets
   a. cong. megakaryocytic hypoplasia (isolated with anomalies)
   b. inherited thrombocytopenia (Wiskott-Aldrich, May-Hegglin)
   c. congenital leukemia and histiocytosis
   d. drugs
3. Both decreased production and increased destruction
   a. cong. infections (toxoplasmosis, rubella, cytomegalovirus herpesvirus, syphilis)
   b. osteopetrosis
4. Miscellaneous
   a. thrombotic thrombocytopenic purpura
   b. inherited metabolic disorders
   c. congenital thyrotoxicosis

These mechanisms can be evaluated by an investigation of the size and appearance of the megakaryocytes in bone marrow samples or platelets in peripheral blood smears.

Determination of platelet survival time by Chromium-51 labelled platelets is technically difficult in the newborn but the response to a transfusion of normal platelets may also give some information about platelet production or destruction.

In neonatal intensive care units thrombocytopenia is mostly found in sick neonates, especially in the low and very low birthweight infants, and associated with many acquired disorders. But thrombocytopenia is also frequently seen in apparently healthy fullterm and premature infants. The most common causes of neonatal thrombocytopenia seen in a neonatal intensive care unit are congenital infections and disseminated intravascular coagulation syndrome (DIC) in a group of sick neonates and immune disorders in a group of apparently healthy neonates.

INFECTIONS

Most specific perinatal infections may be accompanied by thrombocytopenia: e.g., congenital rubella, cytomegalic inclusion disease, toxoplasmosis, syphilis and disseminated herpes simplex infection. Mechanisms for the thrombocytopenia of several congenital infections include hypoplasia of megakaryocytes, increased platelet destruction by splenomegaly and reticuloendothial hyperactivity, and in some instances DIC,[18] although this phenomenon is mostly associated with bacterial septicaemia.

Most of these infants with congenital infections are small for gestational age with hepatosplenomegaly, jaundice and purpura. Laboratory findings give evidence of haemolytic anaemia, thrombocytopenia and hepatitis.

Increased levels of IgM in cord blood support the diagnosis of congenital infection. Therapy should be directed at the underlying infection. Bleeding tendency due to thrombocytopenia is unusual, and when present complication by DIC should be suspected.

DISSEMINATED INTRAVASCULAR COAGULATION SYNDROMES

DIC is a pathological process in which a number of triggering mechanisms cause generation of procoagulants, endothelial damage of small vessels or tissue factor release in the circulation resulting in a generalised consumption of platelets, antithrombin, clotting factors V, VIII, II, XIII and fibrinogen within the circulation.[11,18] Secondary fibrinolysis results in increased amounts of circulating fibrin-fibrinogen degradation products.

Intravascular fibrin deposition leads to microangiopathic erythrocytic changes and to widespread microthrombi with organ dysfunction. Sometimes a thrombotic tendency can occur with large vessel thrombosis and progressive gangrene.[17] Generalised haemorrhage or localised organ bleeding commonly occurs.

DIC probably accounts for most cases of bleeding tendency in sick newborns in whom physiological immunity of clotting pathways, reduced antithrombin levels and impaired reticuloendothelial clearance are contributing factors.[8]

There are many fetal and neonatal disorders in which trigger mechanisms may activate the coagulation system[9] (Table III). Injury to the endothelial vessel wall may activate the intrinsic coagulation system. Release of tissue factor may activate the extrinsic coagulation system. Injury to red blood cells or platelets may accelerate blood coagulation due to release of procoagulant phospholipids, while reticuloendothelial dysfunction may decrease the clearance of activated coagulation factors. The disorders associated with these pathological processes frequently occur in premature infants.

TABLE III

AETIOLOGIC FACTORS IN NEONATAL DIC

1. Activation of intrinsic coagulation system by injury of endothelial vessel wall
   - sepsis, infections, acidosis, hypoxaemia, hyperviscosity, hypothermia, giant haemangioma, indwelling catheters
2. Activation of extrinsic coagulation system by release of tissue factor
   a. obstetric complications - abruptio placentae, eclampsia, dead twin fetus, placental chorangioma, small for gestational age infants, postmature infants
   b. organ necrosis - necrotising enterocolitis, thrombosis
   c. brain injury, surgical procedures, fetal neoplasms
3. Acceleration of blood coagulation by release of phospholipids by injury of red blood cells or platelets
   a. intravascular haemolysis - erythroblastosis fetalis, incompatible RBC transfusion
   b. antigen-antibody reactions
4. Decreased clearance of activated coagulation factors by injury of reticuloendothelial system
   - RES hypofunction, hepatic disease

In bacterial septicaemia thrombocytopenia is commonly present, but the role of DIC is not always evident. It seems that laboratory evidence of DIC is mostly found in proven bacterial septicaemia when platelet counts are less than 50,000 per µl and little or no evidence when platelet counts are 50,000 to 150,000 µl.[34] Because of decreased platelet survival it has been suggested that subclinical or compensated DIC might be a contributing factor in these cases.

It is known that bacterial endotoxin can produce thrombocytopenia without eliciting DIC, suggesting a primary injury of platelets.[10] Diagnosis of DIC is established when platelet counts are less than 150,000 per ml, anaemia persists, Burr cells are seen in peripheral blood smears and fibrinogen levels of less than 150mg/100 ml exist. Levels of factors V and VIII should be less than 50% and fibrinogen split products should be found.

There is general agreement that treatment of DIC must be directed towards the underlying diseases, but specific therapeutic approaches of DIC in the newborn period are still controversial (Table IV). There are no controlled prospective studies comparing various forms of therapy.[25] In a recent retrospective study of 53 cases of DIC in the newborn, by William Woods in 1979,[40] no difference was found in coagulation response or in mortality among patients treated with either fresh frozen plasma, factor concentrates, exchange transfusion, heparin or no treatment.

TABLE IV

THERAPEUTIC APPROACHES IN DIC

1. Administration of platelets and coagulation factors	
a. fresh platelet concentrates	10 ml/kg every 12-24 hr
b. fresh frozen plasma	10-15 ml/kg every 12-24 hr
2. Exchange transfusion with fresh whole blood	180 - 200 ml/kg
3. Heparin	50 units kg loading dose
	10-20 units/kg/hr continuous

There is no controlled clinical evidence for the value of heparin in newborns with DIC.[41] Numerous problems have been found with the use of heparin: heparin-induced thrombocytopenia, heparin inactivity by reduced levels of antithrombin and the release of platelet factor 4 during the consumptive process, difficulty in monitoring the effect of heparin and difficulty with dosage requirements. Perhaps heparin could be indicated in the presence of thrombosis, as in purpura fulminans.

Exchange transfusions with fresh whole blood could be useful in:

1. removing toxins, fibrinogen split products and damaged erythrocytes
2. achieving anticoagulation
3. providing platelets and coagulation factors
4. decreasing tissue hypoxia by replacing fetal haemoglobin with adult haemoglobin, which has a decreased oxygen affinity.

The reported cases, however, are few and the results are different.

The disadvantages of exchange transfusion in these sick, mostly very low birthweight infants are: metabolic derangement, the use of indwelling catheters and possible increased risk of retrolental fibroplasia associated with a decreased oxygen affinity of adult haemoglobin.

Although we prefer fresh heparinised blood for exchange transfusion it could make the bleeding worse in cases of DIC with severe thrombocytopenia. Perhaps the use of fresh CPD blood should be considered in that event.

Fresh platelet concentrates and fresh frozen plasma have been found to improve the clinical situation in infants with DIC[14] although it would seem to be "adding fuel to the fire". Mortality is high among newborn infants with DIC, especially among high-risk, stressed premature infants with low Apgar scores.[25]

IMMUNE THROMBOCYTOPENIA

When generalised petechiae or mucosal bleeding appear in apparently healthy neonates within 48 hours after birth, immune thrombocytopenia should be considered. In such a case PT and PTT will be normal for age, but platelet counts will be moderately or markedly reduced. Thrombocytopenia is the result of neonatal platelet destruction by maternal IgG antibodies crossing the placental barrier. These antibodies are platelet-specific, coating the neonatal platelets and leading to their destruction by the reticulo-endothelial system.

Two types of neonatal immune thrombocytopenia should be distinguished depending on formation: isoimmune and autoimmune.

1. Isoimmune neonatal thrombocytopenia (INT): In INT antibodies are formed by the mother against specific antigens on the infant's platelets which are lacking on her own platelets. The specific platelet antigenetic system most commonly associated with INT is called Zw, with the corresponding antigens Zw^a [29] and Zw^b.[45] This system appears to be that described by Shulman in 1961 as the PL^a system.[39] Other systems found are Ko with Ko^a and Ko^b antigens[41] and BaK with BaK^aantigen[26] (Table V). Only 2-3% of the population is negative for the Zw^aantigen,[29,39] and it is estimated that the frequency of INT is about 1-2 per 10,births.[39]

Clinical manifestations are generally not serious and restricted to petechiae, purpuric spots, melena, haematuria and oozing from the umbilical cord and from needle punctures. Serious thrombocytopenia, however, may cause intracranial haemorrhage during vaginal delivery[40] or even in utero.[49] These haemorrhages account for the high mortality rate of about 13% given in some reviews of this subject.[37]

TABLE V

ANTIGENIC SYSTEM IN ISOIMMUNE THROMBOCYTOPENIA

System	Antigen	Genotype	Fenotype	Frequency	Antibody
Zw (Pl)	Zw^a (Pl^{a1})	Zw^aZw^a	Zw^a-pos	97.6%	anti-Zw^a (IgC)
		Zw^aZw^b			
	Zw^b (pl^{a2})	Zw^bZw^a			
		Zw^bZw^b	Zw^a-neg	2.4%	anti-Zw^b (IgM)
Ko	Ko^a	Ko^aKo^a	Ko^a-pos	14.3%	anti-Ko^a (IgM)
		Ko^aKo^b			
	Ko^b	Ko^bKo^a			
		Ko^bKo^b	Ko^a-neg	85.7%	anti-Ko^b (IgM)
Bak	Bak^a				

In mild thrombocytopenia, no therapy is needed. The therapy of choice in severe bleeding is transfusion of platelets that lack the responsible antigens.

Since nearly 98% of the general population is Zw^a positive administration of random donor platelets is not effective. Because the mother is negative for this antigen, maternal plateletpheresis and transfusion of these platelets after washing them with plasma is the most effective therapy.[2,31]

Thrombocytopenia may reoccur after some days but bleeding is rarely seen after a week. Generally the thrombocytopenia will last for some days, or even weeks, in both treated and non treated cases. Corticosteroids have been recommended[2,37] but have never been proved convincingly to alter the course of thrombocytopenia. They may well be effective in establishing vascular wall integrity by inhibition of prostacycline generation by the vessel wall.[5] In cases with very low platelet counts or actual bleeding, exchange transfusion to remove antibodies only appears successful when maternal platelets are given directly afterwards.

In any case of INT, all subsequent pregnancies should be considered at risk and careful obstetric management offered. To diminish risk of intracranial haemorrhage during vaginal delivery, caesarian section has been advocated.[40]

TABLE VI

DIFFERENCES BETWEEN ISOIMMUNE AND AUTOIMMUNE

NEONATAL THROMBOCYTOPENIA

	Iso	Auto
Platelet Antigen	specific (Zw^a)	non specific
Platelet Antibody	specific	non specific
Maternal Thrombocytopenia	no	yes*
Neonatal Thrombocytopenia		
- at birth	moderate-severe	moderate
- after some days	severe	severe
Duration of Thrombocytopenia	days-weeks	weeks-months
Clinical Appearances	usual severe	moderate
Therapeutic Effects		
- corticosteroids	doubtful	doubtful
- exchange transfusion	doubtful	doubtful
- random donor platelets	no	no
- maternal platelets	yes	no

*could be normal after splenectomy

----

2. Autoimmune neonatal thrombocytopenia (ANT): In maternal immune thrombocytopenic purpura (ITP) antibodies are formed against the mother's own platelets. In pregnant women with chronic ITP, these antibodies - of the IgG class - may cross the placental barrier and cause transient neonatal thrombocytopenia after birth. In some reports[43,44] the incidence of neonatal thrombocytopenia is supposed to be connected with the state of maternal disease with a high incidence when maternal platelet counts are less than 100,000 per µl and a much lower incidence when platelet counts are more than 100,000 per µl. It should be emphasised, however, that splenectomised women may have normal platelet counts yet still circulate antibodies that will cross the placenta.

It is also possible for antibodies to be of the IgM class and not able to cross the placenta.[27]

It is possible to detect autoimmune and isoimmune antibodies by the platelet suspension immunofluorescence test in which non-specific fluorescence can be prevented by fixing the platelets with paraformaldehyde.[7] Clinical manifestations of ANT as the same as those of INT, although usually less severe, with moderate thrombocytopenia on the first day after birth falling to lower values within some days and lasting some weeks or some months (Table VI).

Comparing the different reviews, an overall perinatal mortality rate is found of about 11%, half of it caused by intracranial haemorrhage.[15,20,25,35]

Most cases of ANT need no other therapy than careful obstetric management. Corticosteroids late in pregnancy seem to improve maternal platelet counts but have no effect on neonatal platelet counts. The benefits of corticosteroids in the neonatal period are still in doubt.

Transfusion of platelets and exchange transfusions have little effect in ANT but should be attempted in cases of serious bleeding. To prevent intracranial haemorrhage, delivery by caesarian section has been advocated.[44]

REFERENCES

1. Aballi, A.: Platelet counts in thriving premature infants. Pediatrics, 42:685, 1968.
2. Adner, M.M. et al: Use of compatible platelet transfusions in the treatment of congenical isoimmune thrombocytopenic purpura. New Engl.J.Med. 280:244, 1969.
3. Appleyard, W.J. et al: Venous platelet counts in low birthweight infants. Biol.Neon. 17:30, 1971.
4. Bell, W.R. et al: Thrombocytopenia occurring during the administration of heparin. Ann.intern.Med. 85:155, 1976.
5. Blajchman, M.A. et al: Shortening of the bleeding time in rabbitis of prostacycline generation by the vessel wall. J.clin.Invest. 63:1026, 1979.
6. Bleyer, W.A. et al: The development of hemostatis in the human fetus and newborn infant. J.Pediat. 79:838, 1971.
7. Borne, A.E.G.Kr.v.d., et al: A simple immunofluorescence test for the detection of platelet antibodies. Brit.J.Haemat. 39:195, 1978.
8. Chessels, J.M. Bleeding problems in the newborn infant. Prog.Hemostasis Thromb. 2:333, 1974.
9. Colman, R.W.: DIC: An approach. Amer.J.Med. 52:679, 1972.
10. Corringan, J.: Thrombocytopenia: A laboratory sign of septicemia in infants and children. J.Pediat. 85:219, 1974.
11. Deykin, D.: The clinical challenge of DIC. New Engl.J.Med. 283:636, 1970.
12. Ekelund, H. et al: Fibrinolysis in newborns. Acta paediat.scand. 59:33, 1970.
13. Fogel, B.J. et al: Platelet counts in healthy premature infants. J.Pediat. 73:108, 1969.
14. Glader, B.E. et al: The bleeding neonate. Pediatrics 58:548, 1976.
15. Goodhue, P.A. et al: ITP in pregnancy. Obstet.Gynec.Surv. 28:671, 1973.
16. Gross, S.J. et al: Haemostasis in the Premature Infant. Clinics in Perinatology. Saunders, vol.4, no.2, 1977.
17. Hathaway, W.E.: The bleeding newborn. Ser.Haematol. 12:175, 1975.
18. Hathaway, W.E.: DIC in the newborn. Pediatrics, 43:233, 1969.
19. Hendriksson, P. et al: Factor XIII in the fetus and the newborn infant. Ped.Rev. 8:789, 1974.
20. Heys, R.F.: Childbearing and ITP. J.Obstet.Gynaec.Brit.Cmwlth, 73:205, 1966.

21. Hilgartner, M.W. et al: Factor XI in the neonate. J.Pediatrics 66:747, 1965.

22. Holmberg, L. et al: Coagulation in the human fetus. Comparison with term newborn infants. J.Pediat. 85:860, 1974.

23. Hrodek, O.: Blood platelets in the newborn. Acta Univ.Carol., 22, 1966.

24. Jensen, A.H. et al: Evaluation of blood clotting factor levels in premature infants during the first ten days of life. Ped.Rev. 7:638, 1973.

25. Laros, R.K. et al: Management of ITP during pregnancy. Amer.J.Obstet.Gynec. 122:182, 1975.

26. Leeuwen, E.F.v. et al: Neutropenie en thrombocytopenie van de pasgeborene, veroozaakt door allo-antistoffen. Ned.T.Geneesk. 124:393, 1980.

27. Leeuwen, E.F.v. et al: Neonatal alloimmune thrombocytopenia complicated by maternal autoimmune thrombocytopenia. Brit.med.J. 281:27, 1980.

28. Levine, P.H.: Platelet function test: Predictive value. New Engl.J.Med. 292:1346, 1975.

29. Loghem, J.J.v. et al: Serological and genetical studies on a platelet antigen (Zw). Vox Sang. 4:161, 1959.

30. Mahasandana, C. et al: Circulating anticoagulants in the newborn: Relation to hypercoagulability and the idiopathic respiratory distress syndrome. Ped.Rev. 7:670, 1973.

31. McIntosh, L.S. et al: Transfusions of antigenically compatible platelets for therapy and diagnosis of isoimmune neonatal thrombocytopenia. Ped.Rev. 6:108, 1972.

32. Medoff, H.S.: Platelet counts in premature infants. J.Pediat. 64:287, 1974.

33. Mull, M. et al: Altered platelet function in newborns. Ped.Rev. 4:229, 1970.

34. Neame, P.B. et al: Thrombocytopenia in septicemia: the role of disseminated intravascular coagulation. Blood, 56:88, 1980.

35. Norriega-Guerra, L. et al: Pregnancy in patients with autoimmune thrombocytopenic purpura. Am.J.Obstet.Gynec. 15:439, 1979.

36. Nossel, H.L. et al: A study of coagulation factor levels in women during labour and in their newborn infants. Thrombosis et Diathesis Haemorrh. 16:185, 1966.

37. Pearson, H.A. et al: Isoimmune neonatal thrombocytopenic purpura: Clinical and therapeutic considerations. Blood, 123:154, 1964.

38. Sell, E.J. et al: Platelet counts, fibrinogen concentration and Factor V and Factor VIII levels in healthy infants according to gestational age. J. Pediat. 82:1028, 1973.

39. Shulman, N.R. et al: Immunoreactions involving platelets. J.clin.Invest. 40:1597, 1961.

40. Sitar, A.L. et al: Management of isoimmune neonatal thrombocytopenia. Amer.J.Obstet.Gynec. 124:39, 1976.

41. Straub, P.W.: A case against heparin therapy of intravascular coagulation. Throm.Diath.Haemorrh. 33:107, 1974.

42. Stuart, M.: Storage pool deficiency in neonatal platelets. Ped.Rev. 11:481, 1977.

43. Tancer, L.M.: Idiopathic thrombocytopenic purpura and pregnancy. Amer.J.Obstet.Gynec. 79:148, 1960.

44. Territo, M. et al: Management of autoimmune thrombocytopenia in pregnancy and in the neonate. Obstet. and Gynec. 41:579, 1973.

45. Weerdt, Ch.M.v.d.: Platelet antigens and isoimmunization. Thesis, Amsterdam, 1965.

46. Whaun, J.M.: The platelet of the newborn infant: 5-hydroxytryptamine uptake and release. Throm.Diath.Haemorrh. 30:327, 1973.

47. Whaun, J.M. et al: The platelet of the newborn infant: Aggregation and adenine nucleotide release. Ped.Rev. 8:41, 1974.

48. Woods, G.W. et al: DIC in the newborn. Amer.J.Dis.Child. 133:44, 1979.

49. Zalneraitis, E.L. et al: Intracranial haemorrhage in utero as a complication of isoimmune thrombocytopenia. J.Pediat. 95:611, 1979.

----

2. CYTAPHERESIS SUPPORT IN CHILDHOOD ONCOLOGY

A. POSTMA

As of today, survival rates in paediatric oncology have shown a dramatic improvement due to advances in multimodality of treatment. Advances in chemotherapy have made a particular contribution to more effective ways of treating malignant disease in childhood. On the other hand, the increasing role of chemotherapy may result in severe complications to the haematopoietic system. The paediatric oncologist has frequently to deal with disease-induced, and even more often with drug-induced, leucopenia and thrombocytopenia.

There is a clear correlation between the degree of granulocytopenia and the acquisition of bacterial and fungal infections.[4,5] In patients with leukemia, infection remains a leading cause of death.[3,5,7]

Various approaches have been used in an attempt to control infection.[7] It is of common knowledge that preservation of a good nutritional state is of great importance in supporting immunologic capacities.

During episodes of severe immunosuppression, enforced isolation may protect the patient from exogenous infections.[4] Intestinal decontamination plays an important role in the prevention of endogenous infections.[4]

As soon as septicaemia is clinically suspected or established, multidrug and high dose antibiotic therapy must be initiated, preferably with bacteriocidal drugs to which the pathogen is sensitive.[1,3,8] However, this treatment alone may be ineffective in patients with granulocytopenia: in such cases leucocyte transfusion seems a logical treatment.[3,4,5,7]

Thrombocytopenia is a frequent complication in patients with malignant disease, whether as a result of the disease process itself or of the therapy that is administered.

Several investigators have shown that thrombocyte transfusions may be of use in controlling haemorrhage secondary to thrombocytopenia.[2,9] In some institutions it is routine to administer thrombocytes prophylactically to all patients with thrombocytopenia.[6] However, the development of antibodies which interfere with future transfusions is one of the serious risks of the prophylactic use of thrombocytes.[2,6,9] In this paper we evaluate the leucocyte and thrombocyte transfusions administered in our own institution between 1977 and 1979.

We used single donor leucocyte and thrombocyte collections obtained by means of discontinuous flow centrifugation by haemonetic 30 machine. The number of leucocytes per transfusion was 0.6 - 0.9 x 10^{10} and the number of thrombocytes per transfusion 3.2 - 4.8 x 10^{11}. Donors were selected on ABO and rhesus compatibility; there was no selection on the basis of HLA typing. No family donors were used in this period.

Leucocyte Transfusions

From 1977-79, 15 patients, ages 4-16 years, received a total of 73 leucocyte transfusions in 18 episodes. Six of the 15 children had acute leukemia. In suspected infection or septicaemia, samples were taken from the nose, throat, urine, stools and blood and another antibiotic regimen instituted. As a rule, chemotherapy was then stopped, except for those patients in the induction phase of leukemia treatment.

Leucocyte transfusions were administered daily for a minimum of three days, or until the number of peripheral leucocytes increased above 1000/ml and fever reduced. The number of transfusions per episode ranged from 1 to 10. Two patients died on the first and second day respectively after starting leucocyte administration. One patient had 10 consecutive transfusions.

In 10 of the 18 episodes of leucocyte transfusions, the peripheral number of leucocytes rose above 1000/ml. In this group one patient died of pulmonary complications.

No increment of leucocytes was seen in seven episodes. In this group three patients died at the second, the fifth and the sixth day of leucocyte transfusion. One patient died shortly after the first leucocyte transfusion and could not be evaluated.

The isolated pathogens were mainly bacteria belonging to the intestinal flora. In 9 episodes blood cultures were negative. Three patients with positive cultures and two with negative cultures died.

In summary: 18 episodes of suspected or documented infection resistant to antibiotics, in 15 granulocytopenic children, were treated with leucocyte transfusion. Five of the patients died and 10 survived. The role of the leucocyte transfusion is difficult to establish since the effect of natural recovery due to the interruption of chemotherapy must be taken into account.

Bacteriological inventarisation in granulocytopenic patients is becoming more important in the prevention of serious infections. As many of the pathogens responsible originate from the intestinal tract, decontamination might be effective in patients at high risk of bone marrow depression. In our department a decreasing incidence of Gram-negative septicaemia was noticed and consequently the need for leucocyte transfusions decreased.

Thrombocyte transfusions

Our indications for thrombocyte transfusions were thrombocytopenia and haemorrhage or surgical intervention. From 1977-79, 50 patients, ages 3 months to 18 years, received 90 thrombocyte transfusions. Almost half of these patients were suffering from acute leukemia. One patient had a giant haemangioma, a benign conditions with massive consumption of thrombocytes and disturbed coagulation.

Nearly 50% of all thrombocyte transfusions were given for nasopharyngeal bleeding, 10% for retinal haemorrhage with imminent intracranial bleeding and 12% for surgical intervention. If haemorrhage did not stop, a subsequent transfusion was given on the next day. More than 50% of patients showed a thrombocyte increment 24 hours after transfusion above 20,000/ml.

In most cases bleeding stopped following local therapy and administration of thrombocytes. A correlation can be shown between the success of the transfusion and the increment of thrombocytes. But there was no correlation between thrombocyte increment and antibodies against leukocytes. Figures showing the relation between the number of thrombocyte transfusions per patient and antibodies are not conclusive about the cause of sensitisation because many patients had previously received other non irradiated blood components.

One patient died from bleeding. This was a 3-months-old boy with high risk ALL who died from intracranial haemorrhage in the first week of induction therapy. All other patients survived haemorrhagic complications.

In conclusion, we think that thrombocyte transfusion has an important role in supportive care of children treated for malignant disease. The availability of thrombocytes for transfusion will permit chemotherapy to be continued even in cases of thrombocytopenia so that more effective treatment may be offered and a higher survival rate obtained.

Summary

1. Leucocyte transfusions seem to be a useful addition to antibiotic therapy in granulocytopenic patients with bacterial infections.
2. The need for leucocyte transfusions will be decreased by effective preventive measures.
3. Thrombocyte transfusions are valuable in the management of patients with thrombocytopenia.
4. The availability of thrombocyte transfusions permits continuation of chemotherapy despite drug-induced thrombocytopenia.

Acknowledgement

This work could not have been completed without the support of the Red Cross Bloodbank Groningen-Drenthe who also provided the necessary cytapheresis information and statistics.

REFERENCES

1. Alavi,J.B., Root, R.K., Djerassi, I., Evans, A.E., Gluckman, S.J., McGregor, R.R., Guerry, D., Schreiber, A.D., Shaw, J.M., Kock, P. and R.A. Cooper: A randomized clinical trial of granulocyte transfusions for infection in acute leukemia. New.Engl.J.Med. 296:706, 1977.
2. Alvarado, J., Djerassi, J. and S. Farber: Transfusion of fresh concentrated platelets to children with acute leukemia. J.Pediat. 67:13, 1965.
3. Fortuny, I.E., Bloomfield, C.D., Hadlock, D.C., Goldman, A., Kennedy, B.J. and J.J. McCullough: Granulocyte transfusion: A controlled study in patients with acute non-lymphocytic leukemia. Transfusion, 15:548, 1975.
4. Graham Pole, J., Davies, M., Kershaw, I., Barter, D.A.C. and M.L.N. Willoughby: Granulocyte transfusion in treatment of infected neutropenic children. Arch.Dis.Childh. 51:521, 1976.
5. Herzig, R.H., Herzig, G.P., Graw, R.G., Bull,M.I. and K.K. Ray: Successful granulocyte transfusion therapy for Gram-negative septicemia. New Engl.J.Med. 296:701, 1977.
6. Higby, D.J., Cohen, E., Holland, J.F. and L. Sinks: The prophylactic treatment of thrombocytopenic leukemic patients with platelets: A double blind study. Transfusion, 14:440, 1974.
7. Higby, D.G., Freeman, A., Henderson, E.S., Sinks, L. and E. Cohen: Granulocyte transfusions in children using filter collected cells. Cancer, 38:147, 1976.
8. Pizzo, P.A., Ladisch, S. and K. Robichaud: Treatment of Gram-positive septicaemia in cancer patients. Cancer, 45:206, 1980.
9. Van Eys, J., Thomas, D. and B. Olivos: Platelet use in pediatric oncology: A review of 393 transfusions. Transfusion, 18:169, 1978.

----

3. PLATELET TRANSFUSION IN BONE MARROW TRANSPLANTATION IN CHILDREN

J. de KONING

INTRODUCTION

Bone marrow transplantation may lead to a complete recovery in children with aplastic anaemia, acute leukemia and severe combined immunological deficiency. The history of bone marrow transplantation parallels the improvement in transfusion procedures, i.e., the development of blood component therapy. The aim of blood component therapy and of the precautions taken is a fair therapeutic result without isoimmunisation, and avoidance of transfusion-induced graft versus host disease (GVH).

MOMENT OF PLATELET TRANSFUSION

Severe aplastic anaemia is accompanied by a tendency to bleed more or less abundantly. Petechiae, bruises, nasal bleeds and bleeding from other orifices may present. Cerebral and retinal bleedings are extremely alarming. Where these are suspected, platelets should be given immediately. Children with acute leukemia may tend to bleed severely at the moment of diagnosis and during the intensive cytostatic therapy applied to obtain that first complete remission. In aplastic anaemia the need for transfusion is one of the reasons for performing bone marrow transplantation.

Transplantation of bone marrow to children with aplastic anaemia and acute leukemia is only possible if the immunological resistance to transplanted cells is eliminated. The immunosuppressive therapy consists of high dosages of cyclophosphamide, either alone, or in combination with antilymphocyte globulin and procarbazine. Total lymphoid irradiation is of recent usage.

Children with leukemia are pretreated with cyclophosphamide followed by total body irradiation. In leukemia, the remaining leukemic cells are assumed to have been eliminated by this procedure, together with the immunosuppression.

One side effect of pretreatment is an aplasia of all cell lines and damage to the epithelia. This causes bleeding episodes, particularly of the bladder and sometimes of the gut. A high transfusion frequency of red cells and platelet may be used to control these symptoms in the first weeks following the transplantation.

Following a successful transplantation, a recovery of peripheral blood cells should start after two weeks. Generally the erythrocytes and leucocytes recover first, the platelets somewhat later. As a rule, 100 days after transplantation bloodcounts are normal. Repulsion of the transplanted cells results in new aplastic signs and suggests a new transplantation. Acute graft versus host disease is a feared side effect. In this syndrome, an immunological reaction of donor cells with the patient's cells leads to fever, skin erythema with a strong desquamation of the skin, damage of the mucosa of the gut with profuse

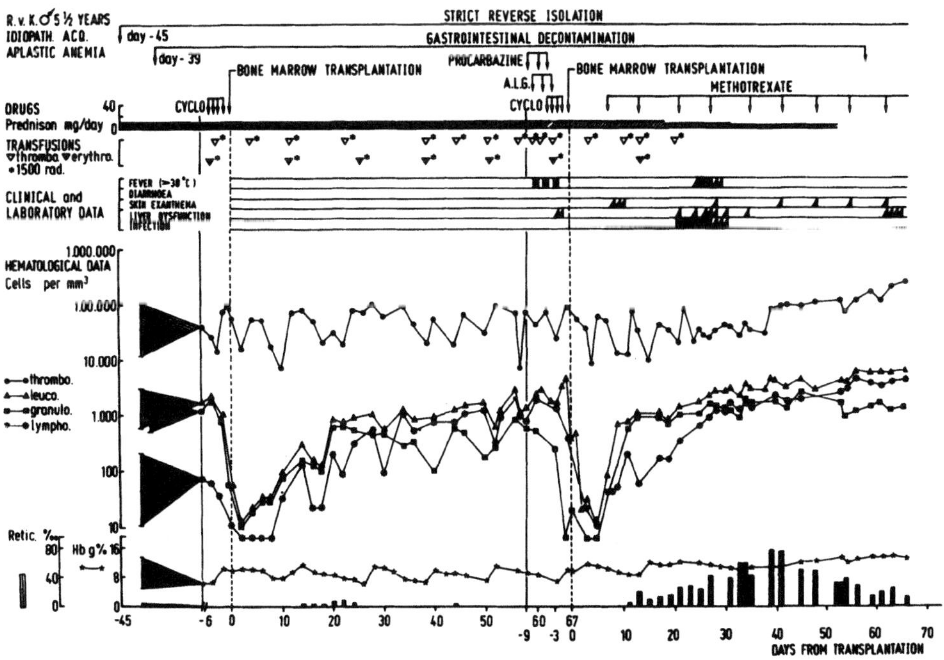

TABLE I

TRANSPLANTATION OF BONE MARROW IN CHILDREN WITH APLASTIC ANAEMIA

Patients/ Age/Sex	Aetiology	Take/GVH		Follow up (months)	Complications
10 yr - M	idiopathic	+	-	84	
6 yr - M	idiopathic	±	-	77	
7 yr - F	idiopathic	+	+	69	
11 yr - M	idiopathic	+	-	50	
15 yr - F	idiopathic	+	-	43	
10 yr - M	idiopathic	+	-	27	
10 yr - M	idiopathic	+	+	22	
8 yr - M	idiopathic	+	±	7	
10 yr - F	idiopathic	-	-		34 d. sepsis
7 yr - F	idiopathic	±	+		25 d. cardiotoxicity CVA, sepsis
12 yr - M	idiopathic	-	-		13 d. cardiotoxicity CVA, sepsis
		-	-		
5 yr - M	idiopathic	+	+		9 months bronchiolitis
10 yr - M	idiopathic	+	-		12 d. sepsis
12 yr - M	idiopathic	+	-		58 d. renal insuff.
16 yr - M	familial	+	++		72 d. GVH
12 yr - F	Fanconi	+	±	57	
10 yr - M	Fanconi	+	++		40 d. GVH
12 yr - F	Fanconi	+	++		38 d. GVH
10 yr - F	Fanconi	+	++		49 d. bleeding of gut & bladder
9 yr - M	hepatitis	+	-	72	
12 yr - M	hepatitis	+	±	80 days	

(Leiden Paediatric Dept. 1980)

diarrhoea and liver function disturbances. In the attempt to treat acute GVH with antilymphocyte globulin, further platelet transfusions are often necessary. The clinical course of a successful bone marrow transplantation of a child with aplasia is presented in Fig. 1. There are many published reports[1,4,8,10] of the results of bone marrow transplantations. While ±50% of children with severe aplastic anaemia may recover completely, poor results are obtained in transplantations of children with Fanconi anaemia.[5] The clinical results of transplantation of children with aplastic anaemia of the Pediatric Department, University of Leiden, are presented in Table I. Of 14 patients with ideopathic aplastic anaemia transplanted, 8 made a complete recovery, but only 1 of the 4 patients with Fanconi anaemia recovered.

Transplantation of patients with aplasia following hepatitis was a success in 2 of 3 cases. One patient with familial aplastic anaemia died. Of the total group of 22 patients, a bone marrow transplantation procured a recovery of the aplastic anaemia in 11 of the patients.[10]

Until recently, the results of bone marrow transplantation in acute leukemia were very disappointing. Transplantation during the first complete remission of acute non-lymphatic leukemia is a new development, and 60-70% leukemia-free survival during more than two years is reported.[7,9] Platelet transfusions, often administered in aplastic anaemia and acute leukemia, are not necessary in severe combined immunological deficiency disease.

PROBLEMS OF PLATELET TRANSFUSION

When platelet transfusions are applied before and during bone marrow transplantation attention has to be paid to:

1. the mechanism leading to thrombocytopenia,
2. the presence of allo - or auto - antibodies
3. the choice of platelet donor,
4. the amount, purification and irradiation of platelet suspensions.

The thrombocytopenia of aplastic anaemia has its origins in a diminished production of platelets. A similar mechanism is present or assumed in the leukemic phase of leukemia, during cytostatic treatment and extensive radiotherapy. Other mechanisms leading to thrombocytopenia are an increased destruction of platelets as in idiopathic thrombocytopenia and an increased consumption of platelets in diffuse intravascular coagulation of infections with Gram-negative microorganism. Massive bleeding leads to loss of platelets. The mechanisms leading to thrombocytopenia are studied with ^{51}Cr thrombocyte survival studies.[6]

The platelet survival time of normal platelets is 8 days. The same platelet survival time is observed in aplastic anaemia. In idiopathic thrombocytopenia, postviral thrombocytopenia and diffuse intravascular coagulation the platelet survival is shortened, sometimes to minutes. This implies that a therapeutic platelet suspension has a better and longer effect if the survival time is expected to be normal and has a less and shorter effect if the survival time is shortened.

During the treatment of aplasia the regular use of transfusions may give rise to alloimmunisation. In rare cases of aplastic anaemia immunisation against platelets is present without a history of previous transfusions of blood and blood products. In these cases an autoimmune disease may be the cause of the aplasia. In Fig. 2 data are presented of two years treatment with platelet transfusions of a 4-year-old girl with aplastic anaemia not responding to conventional treatment. Following the use of HLA non-identical platelets and non-filtered red blood cells, resistance to these platelets suggested the use of paternal and maternal platelets. When resistance to these donors also developed, HLA identical non-related donors were used.

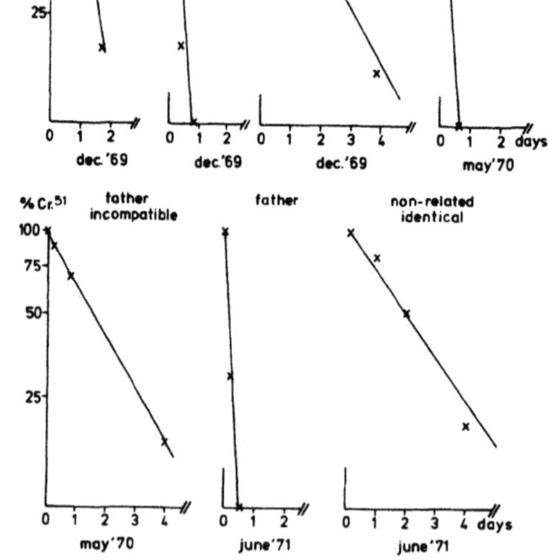

Platelet antibodies are present as a consequence of alloimmunisation or as a result of an autoimmune phenomenon. Alloantibodies arise after one or more transfusions of full blood, granulocyte or platelet suspensions. Alloimmunisation is directed against HLA-specific or platelet-specific antigens.

The detection of these antibodies is complicated. Many different techniques are described for in vitro detection of human antibodies (Table II).

TABLE II

IN VITRO TESTS USED IN PLATELET IMMUNOLOGY

Clot retraction inhibition	Precipitation reaction
Platelet agglutination	Mixed antiglobulin reaction
Platelet lysis	Thrombolastography
Complement fixation	Immunofluorescence
Antiglobulin reaction direct	^{14}C serotonin uptake inhibition
Antiglobulin reaction indirect	Cell electrophoresis
Two Stage agglutination	^{51}Cr release
Passive haemagglutination	Platelet aggression inhibition
Immunophagocytosis	^{131}I Fab - anti F $(ab)_2$ inhibition
Antiglobulin consumption	Immunofluorescence photometry
Mixed cell agglutination	Lymphocytotoxicity (HLA)
Thromboplastin generation inhibition	

The clinical importance of a combination of in vitro tests is presented in Table III. A-match platelet transfusions (donor cells share HLA antigens with the recipient) combined with a negative lymphocytotoxicity test resulted in a 30% failure. With the use of the lymphocytotoxicity test combined with the indirect immunofluorescence test, the results of A-match platelet transfusions are better. The same effect is observed in B-match transfusions (donor and recipient not having incompatible antigens).

The choice of a platelet donor on the basis of HLA typing and in vitro testing is time consuming and complicated. Prevention of alloimmunisation could save a lot of work. The benefit to the patient is a better therapeutic result. Lowering the number of antigenic cells (lymphocytes) may prevent or postpone alloimmunisation.

TABLE III

SELECTION OF PLATELETS ON THE BASIS OF HLA TYPING

AND IN VITRO STUDY OF ANTIBIOTICS

	HLA typed Lymphocytotoxicity test negative		HLA typed Lymphocytotoxicity test negative Indirect platelet immunofluorescence negative	
	RESULTS			
match	fair	poor	fair	poor
A match*	55	23 (30%)	27	1 (3%)
B match*	68	33 (33%)	42	1 (2%)
C match*	24	48 (67%)	18	14 (44%)

*A match: donor and recipient share HLA antigens
B match: donor and recipient have no incompatible antigens
C match: donor and recipient have incompatible antigens

(Brand and Eernisse)[3]

Red cell suspensions filtered via cottonwool filter and lymphocyte-poor platelet suspensions lower the rise of alloimmunisation (Table IV). The amount of platelets transfused is dependent on the age and size of the recipient and the quality of the platelets. In younger children, one to three units of blood produce enough platelets to control bleeding. In older children more units may be necessary. More units are also necessary if the platelets are frozen or derived from blood that is some days old. Patients with aplastic anaemia or leukemia during bone marrow transplantation and children with severe combined immunological deficiency have an impaired cellular immunity. Platelet transfusions and blood transfusions containing viable lymphocytes could give rise to engraftment of these lymphocytes. This carries the danger of graft versus host disease. This danger was described in our first description of an SCID patient.[2] Irradiation of the transfusions with 1200 Rad. kills the lymphocytes without impairment of the function of the platelets.

TABLE IV

LONG TERM TRANSFUSION POLICY
AND POSTPONEMENT OF SENSITIZATION TOWARDS PLATELETS

Before 1974: Red cells without buffycoat platelet concentrates contaminated with leucocytes

After 1974: Filtered+ red cells (without leucocytes)
purified platelet concentrates (without leucocytes)

\+ filtered via filter of Central Laboratory, Dutch Red Cross

		N	%
Before 1974:	refractory	26	93
	non-refractory	2	7
	TOTAL	28	
After 1974:	refractory	16	24
	non-refractory	52	76
	TOTAL	68	

(Brand & Eernisse)[3]

SUMMARY

The platelet transfusion regimen before and during bone transplantation is discussed. Avoidance of alloimmunisation and of graft versus host disease are the principal purposes.

In vitro testing of alloantibodies contributes to a better result of platelet transfusion. In cases of alloimmunisation HLA typing of donor platelets is necessary.

Acknowledgement

The author is indebted to Prof. Dr. L.J. Dooren, Prof. Dr. J.J. Vossen and Dr. R.P. Kamphuis who provided data of bone marrow transplantation, and Dr. J.G. Eernisse and Dr. A. Brand who provided data on platelet immunology.

REFERENCES

1. Camitta, B.M., Thomas, E.D., Nathan, D.G., Santos, G., Gordon-Smith, E.C., Gale, R.P., Rappeport, I.M. and R. Storb: Severe aplastic anemia: A prospective study of the effect of early marrow transplantation on acute mortality. Blood, 48:63, 1976.

2. Dooren, L.J., Vries, M.J.de, Bekkum, D.W.van, Cleton, F.J. and J. de Koning: Sex-linked thymic epithelial hypoplasia in two siblings. J.Pediat. 72:51, 1968.

3. Eernisse, G.J. and A. Brand: Postponement of sensitization against HLA antigens by administration of leucocyte-poor blood components. J.exp.Med.,(in press).

4. Gluckman, E., Devergie, A., Gerotta, I., Hors, J., Sasportes, M., Boiron, M. and J. Bernard: Bone marrow transplantation in 65 patients with severe aplastic anemia. Blut, 41:157, 1980.

5. Gluckman, E., Devergie, A., Schaison, G., Bussel, A., Berger, R., Sohier, J. and J. Bernard: Bone marrow transplantation in Fanconi anaemia. Brit.J.Haemat. 45:557, 1980.

6. Koning, J.de: Diagnostische en therapeutische aspecten van idiopathische thrombocytopenie. Proefschrift Leiden, 1975.

7. Morgenstern, G.R.: Allogeneic bone marrow transplantation for acute leukemia experience in 55 patients. Blut, 41:213, 1980.

8. Santos, G.W., Sensenbrenner, L.L., Burke, P.J., Mullins, G.M., Anderson, P.N., Tutschka, P., Braine, H.G., Davis, T.E., Humphrey, R.L., Abeloff, M.D., Bias, W.B., Borgaonkar, D.S. and R.E. Slavin: Allogenic marrow grafts in man using cyclophosphamide. Transplant.Proc. 6:345, 1974.

9. Thomas, E.D., Buckner, C.D. and A. Fefer: Marrow transplantation in the treatment of acute leukemia. Adv.Cancer Res. 27:269, 1978.

10. Vossen, J.M.J.J., Koning, J.de, Kamphuis, R.P. and L.J. Dooren: Beenmergtransplantatie bij kinderen. Het Medisch Jaar, 1980, p.239.

----

4. DISCUSSION

moderator: N.R.C. ROBERTON

C.Th. SMIT SIBINGA (Groningen, Netherlands): I noted from Dr. de Koning's paper showing the results pre- and post-1974 that the two parameters had been changed: from normal regular red cells to leucocyte-poor red cells, and from normal platelet concentrates to leucocyte-poor platelet concentrates. Can he delineate the results for both of these parameters? What was the actual effect of the leucocyte-poor red cell transfusions on the percentage drop in the immunisation and what is the percentage due to the leucocyte-poor platelet transfusions?

J. de KONING: I have never met such a difficult question! I cannot answer it because we did both at the same time. Looking at the smears of blood with buffycoat there are still 4,000/mm^3 leucocytes present in blood. In cottonwool filtered blood it is much lower. When we made a thrombocyte suspension, which we did from bottles at the time, we went to 1 cm above the line of the buffycoat yet it still contained a lot of lymphocytes. We now take 3 cm or 4 cm above the buffycoat line and see no lymphocytes. If two changes are made at the same time, the effect of each on its own cannot be known. It is known that granulocytes give severe alloimmunisation. We seldom use granulocyte suspensions, but in the few cases when we have, we saw alloimmunisation after one or two transfusions. So I cannot answer the question.

A.S. KHALIFA (Cairo, Egypt): Could Dr. Postma enlarge on her experience of the side effects of leucocyte transfusion. In our experience the patient usually manifests raised temperature, tightness of chest, and sometimes allergic reactions of the skin.

A. POSTMA: All the patients had a raised temperature before we started so that cannot be evaluated. There were no allergic reactions.

S.P. ISRAËLS (Amsterdam, Netherlands): In Amsterdam, the amount of granulocyte concentrates given to patients has been diminishing since the clinicians introduced a method for selective gut decontamination. Has Dr. Postma had a similar experience in Groningen?

A. POSTMA: Possibly the lessening need is because of decontamination, but it is not only due to decontamination. Cultures are better specified and the culture medium is better. We give total decontamination not partial decontamination.

T. GIBSON (Cambridge, U.K.): Which washed solution for platelets did Dr. Bijlmer use?

R.P.G.M. BIJLMER: Washing of platelets is done to remove maternal antibodies from the mother's platelets when we use maternal platelet concentrates. That is why we wash with plasma. We use a solution from normal donor blood and I do not know which precise technology or which procedures are applied by the bloodbank in Nijmegen.

T. GIBSON: The solution we have tried to use in cases where there has been sensitivity to plasma proteins is made up of albumin, 4% glucose and saline. But this is a very infrequent procedure and I wanted to know about the techniques used in Holland.

C.TH. SMIT SIBINGA: I cannot speak for my colleagues from Nijmegen but as far as I know they use autologous plasma; the plasma which comes off the unit.

CONCLUDING REMARKS

J.O. FORFAR

These proceedings of the workshop and symposium will make a significant contribution to our knowledge of bloodtransfusion in paediatrics.

Symposium literally means drinking together. We have been drinking in information, knowledge and understanding of the various disciplines that are represented -

blood transfusion services, paediatrics, obstetrics, microbiology and haematology.

This meeting has brought together in a unique way the laboratory and the ward. It was Dr. Garraty who said that laboratory phenomena should fit clinical findings. I would like to extend that. Laboratory workers and laboratory users should also fit in their understanding of each other.

By meeting together for professional discourse, as we have done, we can make a far more important contribution to the welfare of our patients than if we maintain independence and separateness.

The absence of technical jargon was impressive too, and for that we are indebted to those who so effectively clarified complex subjects, both in their speech and in their diagrammatic presentation.

It was most interesting to hear Dr. Broman, who was a pioneer in the Rhesus field, trace Rhesus problems from the time of his early work up to the present day.

The subject of indications for bloodtransfusion and aspects of such therapy, especially in haemolytic disease of the newborn, has been examined extensively. Dr Roberton raised the controversial issue of the use of heparinised compared with citrated blood. There was no general agreement on this issue, but the opportunity was offered to discuss the pro's and con's. His endorsement of heparinised blood was not something with which the majority seemed prepared to agree, and the balance of opinion appeared to lie with the use of citrated blood.

On this controversial matter, Dr Das's graphical, yet logical plea for the use of citrated rather than heparinised blood in paediatric practice was both impressive and convincing. Clinicians should not ignore that kind of message from a blood transfusion expert and colleague.

Clinical practice cannot be divorced from laboratory realities, and the further we look back, the more clearly we may see how we should move forward. We have not solved all the problems that exist - we hardly expected to do so - but I am sure that we have gone some way to solving some of the problems.

Even more, we have had our eyes opened to problems which up till now we have barely recognised.

The further knowledge and understanding which we have acquired can only improve our practice and allow us to make a more effective contribution in our various professional spheres.

I cannot close without a few final remarks on the way that the conference has been run. I am sure we all applaud the interdisciplinary philosophy behind it, and we have also to applaud the organisation. Conferences do not just happen. They involve an immense amount of planning and work. We are all greatly indebted to Dr. Smit Sibinga and Dr. Das, the staff of the Red Cross Bloodbank Groningen-Drenthe, and all the others who helped them.

The result of their efforts has been a remarkably smooth and effectively organised conference.

GPSR Compliance

The European Union's (EU) General Product Safety Regulation (GPSR) is a set of rules that requires consumer products to be safe and our obligations to ensure this.

If you have any concerns about our products, you can contact us on ProductSafety@springernature.com

In case Publisher is established outside the EU, the EU authorized representative is:

Springer Nature Customer Service Center GmbH
Europaplatz 3
69115 Heidelberg, Germany

Batch number: 10607222

Printed by Printforce, the Netherlands